The
Big Book o
Clinical Research

The Big Book of Clinical Research

A Workbook Containing Puzzles Based on Clinical Research Topics

Crosswords | Jumbled Words | Word Search | Odd-One-Out | Process Flows

Sanjay Gupta

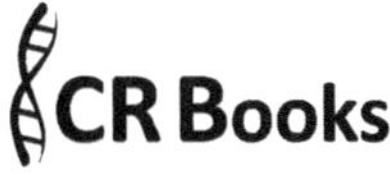

First published in India by
CR Books Pvt. Ltd.
503, Block-C, NDM-2, Netaji Subhash Place, Pitampura, Delhi-110034
Tel. : 011-45121445 Fax : 011-45121435
E-mail : info@crbooks.in, cr.booksltd@gmail.com

First Edition : January 2011

The author and publisher have made a conscientious effort to ensure that the information contained in this book is accurate and in accordance with the accepted standards at the time of publication. However, in this rapidly changing world guidelines and practices are subject to change without prior notification, therefore readers are advised to confirm these as and when needed.

Printed and bound by Elite Printer
eliteprinter@yahoo.in

ISBN 81-908277-2-0

Contents

List of Contributors vi

Preface vii

1. Crosswords 1
2. Jumbled Words 152
3. Word Search 167
4. Odd-One-Out 199
5. Process Flows 208

List of Contributors

1. Dr. Piyush Juneja
2. Gaurav Goel
3. Dr. Ashish Khanduri
4. Dr. Sriram Inamdar
5. Dr. Lokesh Behal
6. Mohd. Nabid

Preface

Clinical Research is an indispensable component of the new drug development process to ensure that the drug, which is to be marketed, is safe and effective. Typically it takes 10-12 years and millions of dollars to bring one new drug to the market with a very limited success rate. Being a highly specialized job function, it requires specific skill-sets to carry out various operations. These involve knowledge about clinical trial processes, standards governing clinical research, regulatory framework etc. Due to the lack of application of all the acquired knowledge on clinical research to the real-time projects, one always have dilemma about his/her competence level.

This book is a unique resource guide on clinical research with inbuilt provision of hands on training. It is intended to serve as a workbook for fun learning through crosswords, jumbled words, word search, odd-one-out and process flows based on clinical research topics. It provides an opportunity to evaluate the competency level of a person regardless of his/her job level.

I hope the book would leave the desired impression and look forward to receive the feedback from the readers at sanjay@catalystclinicalservices.com

12th January 2011 Sanjay Gupta

1

Crosswords

In this section you will find **150** Crosswords containing 12 questions each (across and down). You have to use the clues mentioned below the crosswords for completing the individual crossword. The solution should fill all the boxes (either across or down) mentioned after the individual number.

Please note that the solutions could be,

i. A single word (e.g. Site) or multiple words (e.g. Site Initiation),
ii. A widely used abbreviation of the original term,
iii. A numeral,
iv. A numeral to be specified in words etc.

Scoring: Excellent (able to solve ≥135 crosswords); Very Good (≥120 to <135 crosswords); Good (≥105 to <120 crosswords); Satisfactory (≥75 to <105 crosswords); Unsatisfactory (<75 crosswords).

P
H
A
S
E
1

Across

3. Health service offered on outpatient basis without requiring hospitalization.
5. Safety reporting of marketed drugs in a specified period of time (generally on an annual basis).
6. IND application form.
8. The branch of medical science that deals with the study of incidence, distribution and control of a disease in a population.
11. Central value from a series of observation around which all other observations are dispersed.
12. Assessment of adverse events and serious adverse events experienced by the participants in a clinical trial.

Down

1. Trial phase that evaluates the initial safety of a drug product.
2. Refers to the amount of a drug product to be administered at each specific dosing time.
4. Measurements taken usually at the beginning of a study to serve as a reference for subsequent measurements.
7. The year in which Schedule Y of drug and cosmetics act was introduced.
9. Therapeutic area for which phase 1 clinical trial are conducted on patients rather than healthy volunteers.
10. A drug discovery approach that involves testing the potential drug substances against the target using automated robotic techniques.

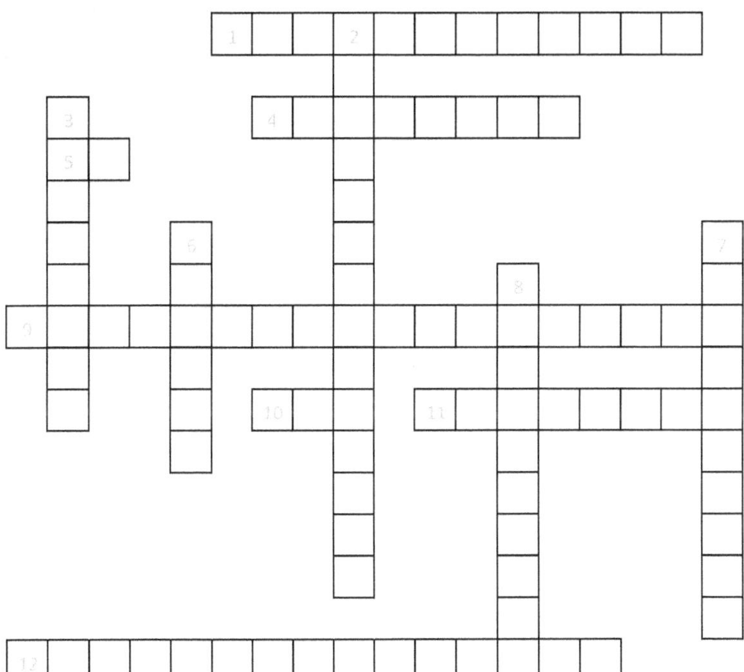

Across

1. A preventive measure.
4. Personal capacity to make choices, consider alternatives and act without undue influence or interference of others.
5. Guidelines for the structure and content of clinical study reports.
9. Methods and strategy used to determine the point at which the overall study data will be considered validated.
10. Drug Regulatory Agency in USA.
11. A brief summary including the objectives, methods, results and conclusion of a clinical trial or any other research work.
12. Biological timing and rythmicity that in human beings is characterized by cycles of approximately 24 hours.

Down

2. Documents given to subjects for recording certain observations on the condition of their health, at their home or at trial site.
3. A pre-designed form/document that includes standard fill-in-the-blank spaces for capturing the standard information.
6. Tests conducted inside the body of a living organism.
7. Review of facility and resources are the critical elements of clinical trial.
8. An independent personnel or organization, hired for performing a specific duty.

Crossword # 3

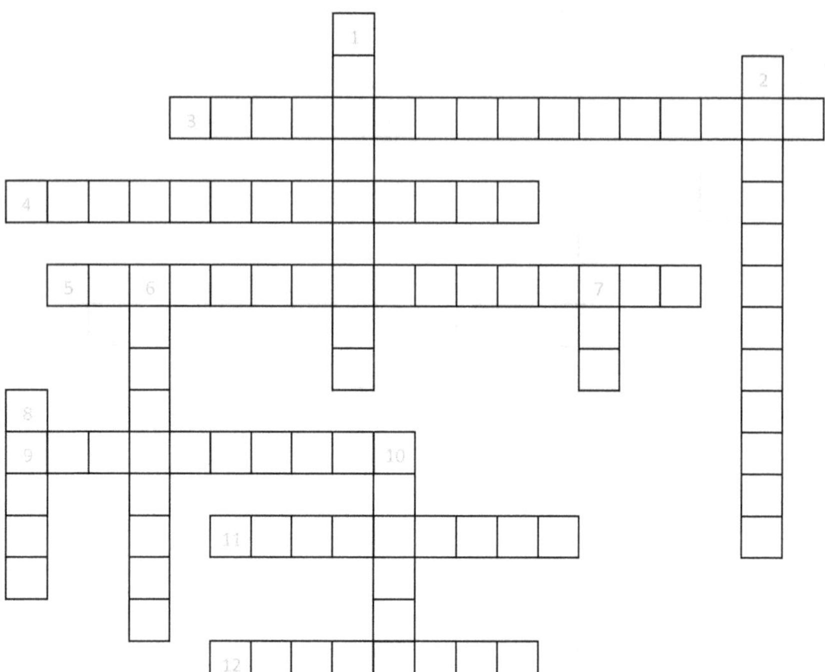

Across

3. Study of genetic variation underlying differential response to drugs.
4. The total number of deaths relative to the total population at a specific place in a specific period of time.
5. LD50/ED50.
9. Scientific rationale of a clinical trial.
11. A law which excludes the users from using original works of authorship, fixed in any tangible medium of expression.
12. The process of absorption, distribution, metabolism and excretion of a drug or a vaccine in a living organism is referred to as Pharmaco________________.

Down

1. Refer to the mock runs for any activity or process, before performing it in a real time environment.
2. An official communication from regulatory bodies to trial sponsor/ investigator/EC documenting its decision.
6. The study of cost-benefit ratio of drugs with other therapies or with similar drugs is known as Pharmaco________________.
7. A document generated to resolve the data query on a particular page of CRF.
8. Average time period(years) for the review of NDA for new molecular entities by FDA.
10. Sequence of instructions that are interpreted or carried out by another program.

Crossword # 4

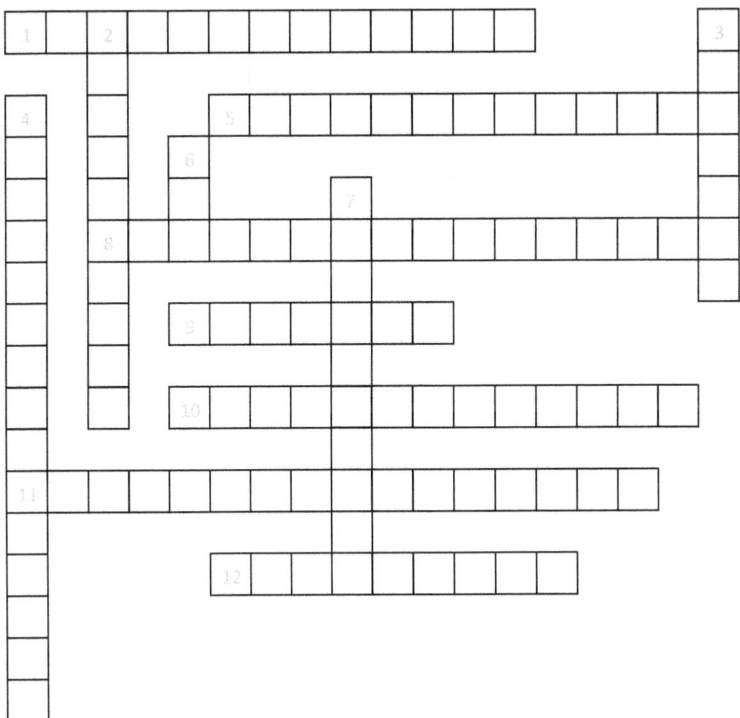

Across

1. Any investigation in human subjects intended to discover or verify the clinical, PK/PD, and adverse reactions of an investigational product.
5. Compounds identified via high throughput screening process.
8. Action letter from the regulatory agency after review of a NDA, which signals that the drug can be approved.
9. Means "I shall please" in latin.
10. A validated data collection form that contains a series of questions to assess an individual's response on a topic/parameter.
11. A biological molecule used as a marker to measure the progress of a disease or effects of a treatment.
12. A subject who has satisfied the entire protocol requirements and is eligible for the safety and efficacy analysis.

Down

2. A state in which a person is no longer able to manage his or her affairs due to physical and mental disability.
3. A coding system for adverse events that allocates each event to a body system and a diagnosis.
4. The initial visit to investigator site by the sponsor/CRO personnel for evaluating the suitability of investigator and facility.
6. The guidelines published by FDA in the year 1997.
7. Refers to the documentation of activities that allows reconstruction of the course of events.

Crossword # 5

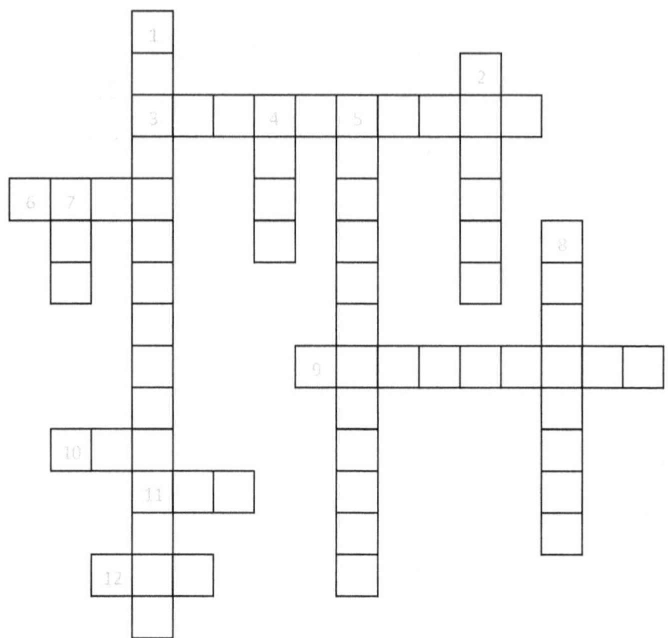

Across

3. Allocation of specific trial related duties to the individual study team members in a clinical trial.
6. ICH topic codes.
9. Type-2 statistical error.
10. Document that establishes agreement between two or more parties for ensuring the confidentiality of information provided by one party to the other.
11. A central file in which all the essential clinical trial documents are filed.
12. An analytical report of a batch of investigational product highlighting its content uniformity and percentage purity.

Down

1. A legal statement or document indicating protection or exemption from liability for compensation or damages from third party.
2. Permission to carry out clinical trials with a new drug in India is issued in _____________.
4. Regulatory agency for regulating clinical trials in Europe.
5. Any untoward medical occurrence in a patient, who has been administered an investigational product and which does not necessarily have a causal relationship with the treatment.
7. Detailed, written instructions to achieve uniformity in the performance of a specific task/activity.
8. A place where drug is prepared and dispensed.

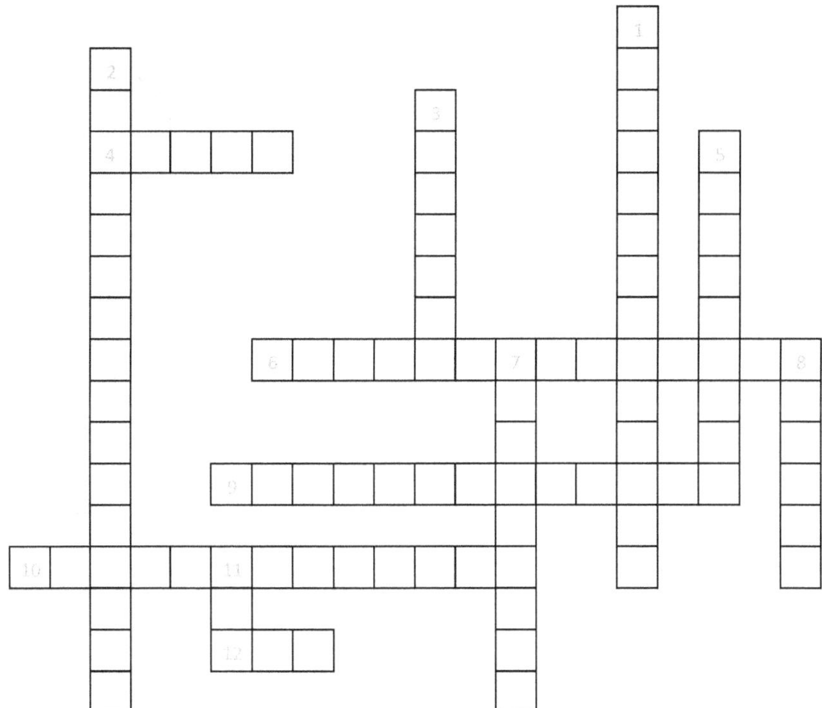

Across

4. A systematic and independent examination to determine whether trial related activities were conducted and the data were recorded, analyzed and accurately reported according to protocol.
6. The arm in a clinical trial refers to ______________.
9. Refer to the subject that does not respond to the trial drug or therapy.
10. A trial design in which subject is randomly assigned to receive either the standard treatment or the investigational drug.
12. A person who assists the investigator in the management of a trial at a site.

Down

1. Refer to organizational hierarchical structure of the supervisors and the subordinates.
2. The processes of absorption, distribution, metabolism, and excretion of a drug or vaccine in a living organism.
3. A part that is a definite fraction of a whole sample for laboratory testing or analysis.
5. Determination of the nature of a disease.
7. The act of signing up participants into a clinical study.
8. First in man studies or trials.
11. An environment in which trial data is directly entered into a web based data management system.

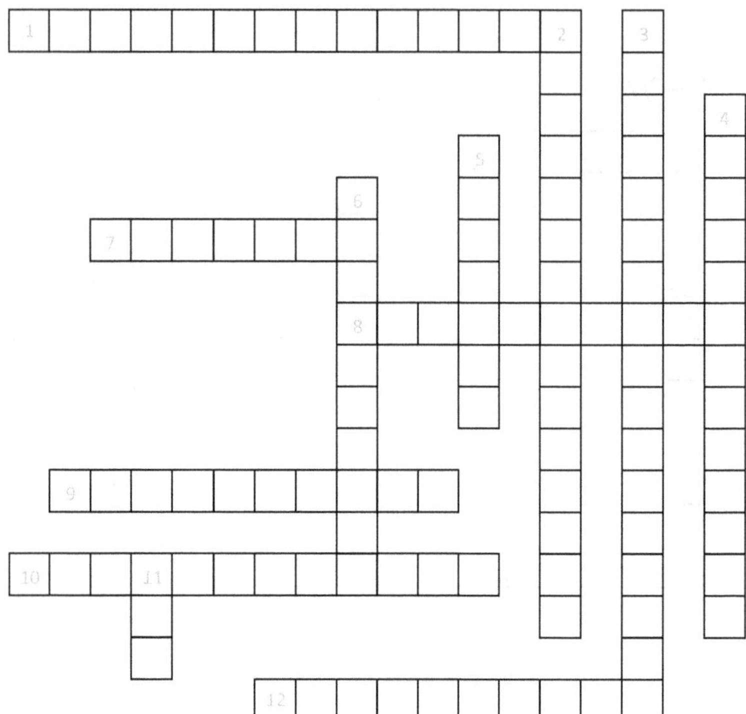

Across

1. An individual, who shares study responsibilities with the investigator at a trial site.
7. The responsibility of the preparation and submission of regulatory dossier lies with ________.
8. The process of evaluation of the hardware and software of a system, to ensure accurate and reliable compliance with user requirements.
9. A set of rules for streamlining processes according to a set routine.
10. Potential of a substance to cause cancer.
12. A substantial disruption of a person's ability to conduct normal life functions.

Down

2. Entry in the electronic case report form using a computer and modem through a distant location.
3. A novel therapy backed by strong scientific data.
4. A result or finding which suggest that an observation is not present but on further investigation is found to be present.
5. Blinding is also known as ________.
6. Refers to the number of people in a given population with a specific condition.
11. Written description of the outcome of a trial.

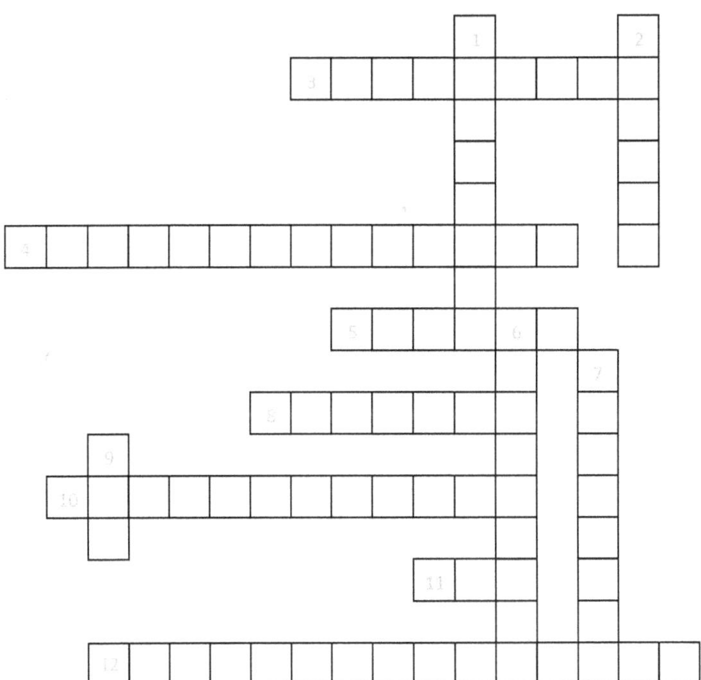

Across

3. The scientific basis or hypothesis of a clinical trial.
4. Documents narrating the conversation or discussion between two or more parties for e.g. letters, emails, fax, telephonic logs etc.
5. Final pre-marketing phase of a clinical trial.
8. Preclinical testing is mainly done on_____________.
10. A person having knowledge and competence of statistics.
11. A classification of regulatory inspection outcome where official action is indicated.
12. Statistical analysis of trial data at a predefined time interval before all subjects has completed the trial.

Down

1. A type of statistical chart that displays information about the distribution of numeric variable.
2. A standardized dictionary of medical terminology adopted by the ICH.
6. Protocol, ICF, IB and CRF constitutes __________clinical trial documents.
7. The study of genetic variation leading to differential response to drugs is called Pharmaco__________.
9. Clinical trial notification is commonly denoted as _______.

Crossword # 9

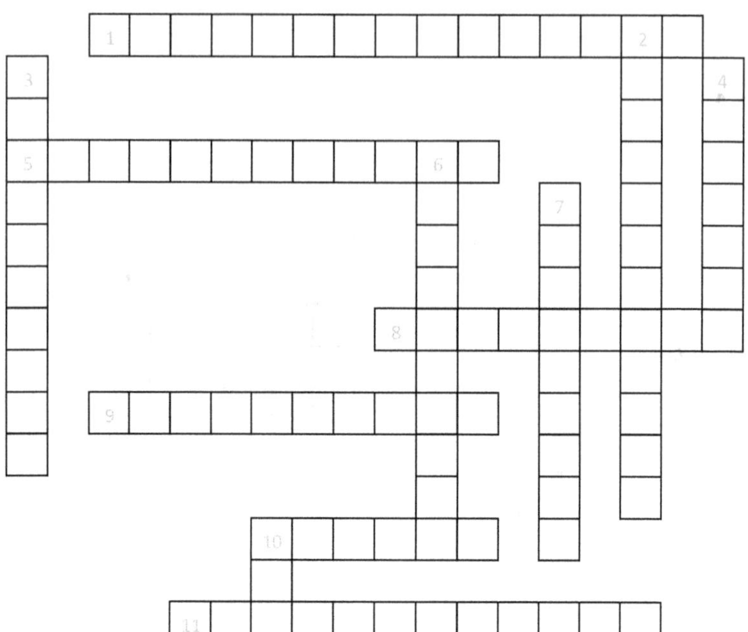

Across

1. Maintaining the minutes of EC meeting is the responsibility of___________.
5. A well controlled, randomized study to evaluate the safety and efficacy of a new drug in patients with relevant disease condition.
8. Pharmaco _____________ refers to methods of assessment and prevention of adverse events.
9. Refers to the relocation of business processes from one country to another.
10. Phase of the trial that involves healthy human volunteers.
11. Supervision of clinical trials by FDA.

Down

2. A log that captures the dates of enrolment and other protocol required visits of a clinical trial subject.
3. Type-1 statistical error.
4. A pattern of black vertical lines containing the coded information to uniquely identify and/or track clinical supplies.
6. Name of a website/web server.
7. A person who submits a trial application to a regulatory agency.
10. A written, dated and signed agreement between two or more parties that sets out arrangements on delegation and distribution of tasks, obligations and if applicable on financial matters.

Crossword # 10

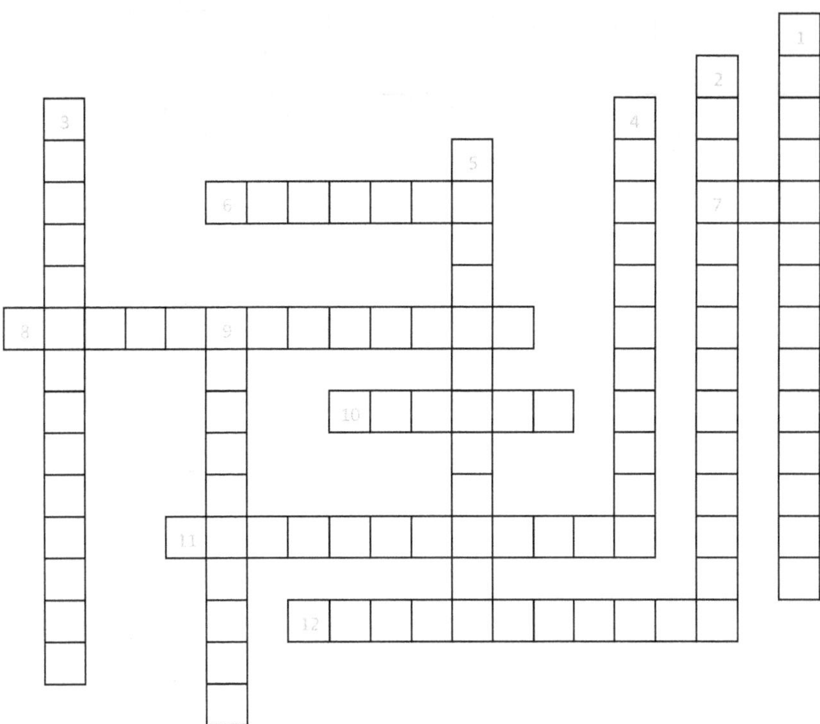

Across

6. A program designed to give supportive care to people in the final phase of a terminal illness either at home, independent facilities or within hospitals.
7. Treatment groups in a randomized trial.
8. Description of the circumstances in which a particular data is required.
10. Phase II of clinical trials evaluates the efficacy and ________.
11. Medical care or payment provided to a subject for trial related injuries.
12. Most effective administration technique if the drug is required to act systematically.

Down

1. Refer to pharmacokinetics of a drug substance.
2. Time frame for reporting serious, unexpected reactions (ADRs) that are not fatal or life-threatening to regulatory agencies as per ICH-GCP (no later than).
3. A medically qualified personnel employed by trial Sponsor/CROs for reviewing critical medical data (safety and efficacy) of a clinical trial.
4. Methodology used to investigate a drug or device for its safety and efficacy.
5. Data to represent situations where the event of interest (e.g. survival, death, response etc.) is not recorded for a patient.
9. An organizational chart that describes different functional positions in an organization.

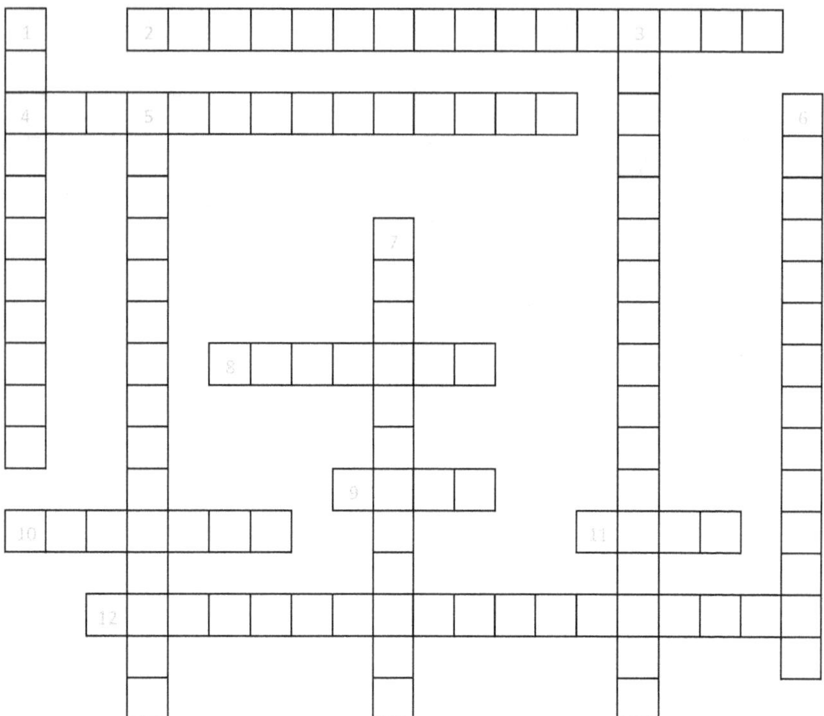

Across

2. Medication taken by a study subject for diseases/medical conditions other than the study disease.
4. A printed, optical, or electronic document designed to record all of the protocol-required information on each trial subject.
8. An individual who participates in a clinical trial either as a recipient of the investigational product or as a control.
9. Animal species on which mutagenicity studies of a new product are conducted.
10. The concentration of a drug at which it is effective.
11. Independent data monitoring committee that may be established by the sponsor, to periodically assess the progress of a clinical trial.
12. An authorization for the use and disclosure of protected health information.

Down

1. US-FDA regulations on financial disclosure by clinical investigators.
3. A person who assists the investigator in the conduct of research project.
5. A procedure by which certain type of research, involving no more than minimal risk, may be reviewed by the chairperson of the ethics committee or designee, without convening a meeting of the entire EC.
6. The process of handling the data collected during a clinical trial.
7. All the SAEs should be personally signed by ___________.

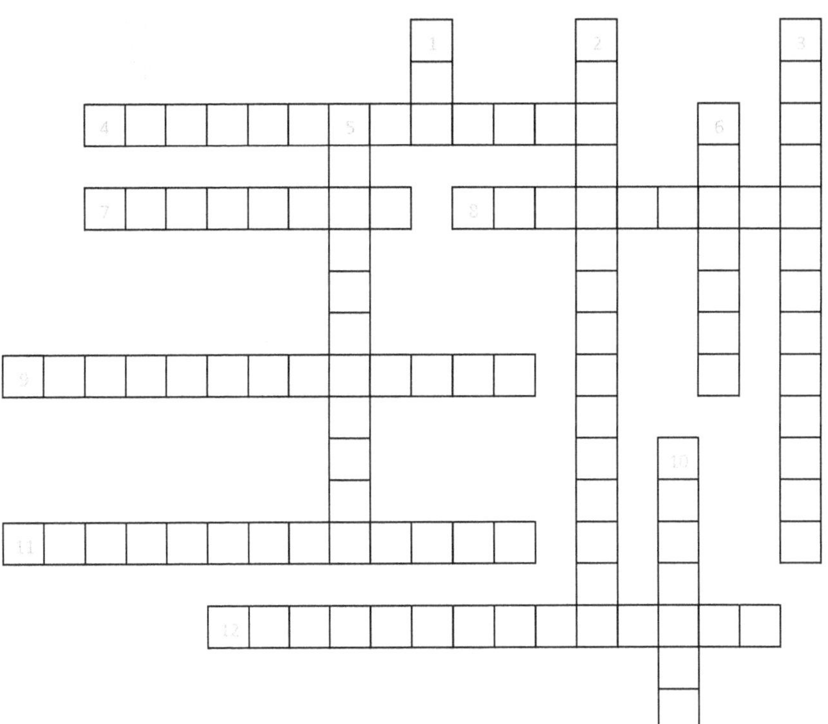

Across

4. Refers to the time period between the initiation and completion of a trial at a site.
7. A dedicated area for the conduct of clinical trials, having required infrastructure and access control facilities.
8. A person who submits a trial application to a regulatory agency.
9. Organization of European countries dedicated to increasing economic integration and strengthening cooperation among its members.
11. A validated data collection form that contains a series of questions to assess an individual's response on a topic/parameter.
12. Information systems for analysis of genomic data.

Down

1. Ethical and scientific quality standards for designing, conducting, recording and reporting trials that involves participation of human subjects.
2. ANDA packet does not include _____.
3. The pieces of information in a clinical trial that have not been recorded even though they should have been collected.
5. Investigator's assessment on the relatedness of an adverse event to the investigational product.
6. An inactive substance designed to resemble the drug being tested.
10. Refer to an observation that is numerically distant from rest of the data.

Crossword # 13

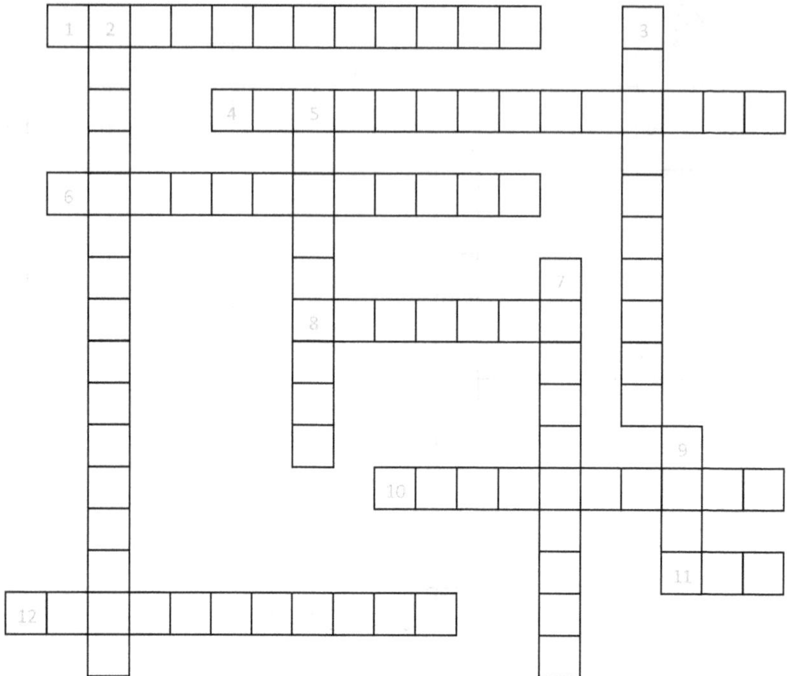

Across

1. A set of patient numbers which are grouped together for statistical purposes.
4. A process of ensuring the accuracy of a clinical trial data using manual checks, computer generated edits, reports or listings.
6. The act of making changes or amendments to an information, document or process.
8. Non clinical testing conducted in an artificial environment (such as a test tube or culture medium).
10. Complexation influences ___ of a drug.
11. ICH Guideline on clinical safety data management.
12. A written plan to define the critical project milestones, cost estimate, timelines and deliverables.

Down

2. A person who has the authority to access and review the trial related documents and activities.
3. An event resulting in death of a subject.
5. Drug Technical Advisory Board is the highest __________ body, under Drug and Cosmetic Act 1940.
7. An agreement between a university and corporate partners for a specific research project or program.
9. Facility for conducting clinical trials.

Crossword # 14

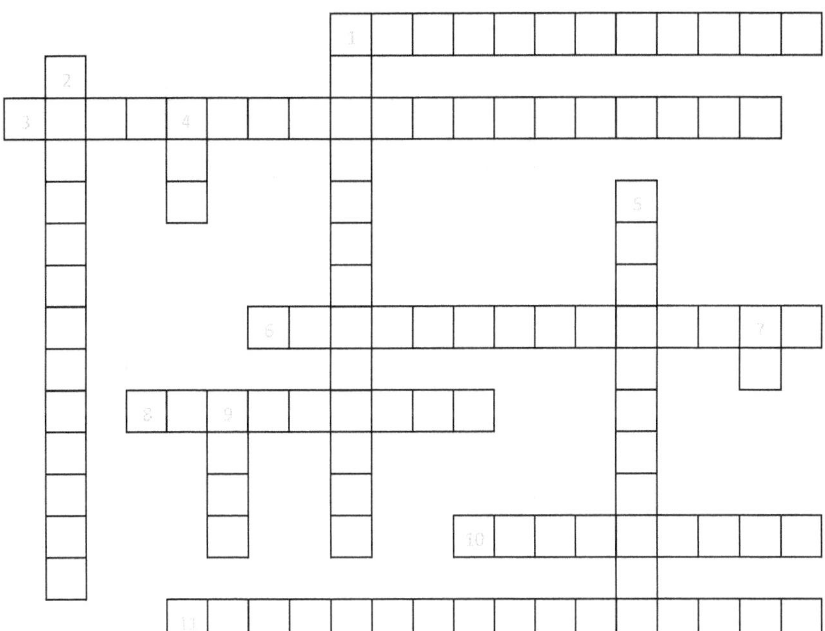

Across

1. A comparison group of study subjects in a trial, who are not treated with the investigational agent.
3. An estimate of survivor function.
6. A patient, who does not meet the inclusion criteria, falls under the category of __________.
8. Refer to the level of fluid in human body.
10. The frequency of disease, illness, injury, and disability in a population.
11. Study of genetic variation leading to differential response to drugs.

Down

1. Statistical test to determine whether there is an association between two categorical variables.
2. A study in which a particular type of subject is equally represented in each study group.
4. Refers to legislation.
5. Disaster that lead to Kefauver Harris Amendment of 1962.
7. Guidelines for statistical principles.
9. A comparison of CRF and ancillary data to the raw data in the clinical trial reporting database.

Crossword # 15

Across

2. A type of drug dosage form used for achieving immediate action.
7. A systematic and Independent examination of trial related activities and documents.
9. The responsibility of filing NDA (New Drug Application) to the regulatory authorities lies with _________.
10. The regression of a disease condition.
11. The ability to understand the purpose, procedures, risks, benefits and alternatives to a research study.
12. Investigation of the pharmacological activity of a new compound using a wide array of chemical and biochemical assays, cell culture models and animal models in a laboratory.

Down

1. Refers to an individual who is legally authorized to consent on behalf of a child for participation in a clinical trial.
3. Longitudinal studies in which the sample is a cohort.
4. An estimate of the total cost implication for carrying out a particular activity.
5. Trial design in which a special type of multi-arm trial allows more than one comparison to be carried out, without increasing the required sample size.
6. A list of commitments and requirements by the FDA, for each investigator performing drug/ biologic studies.
8. A document that describes the objective(s), design, methodology, statistical considerations and organization of a trial.

Crossword # 16

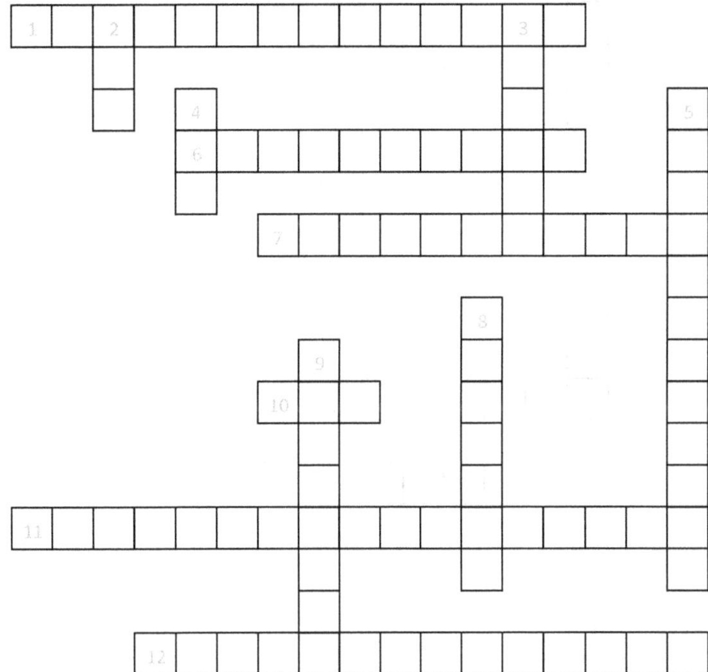

Across

1. Hit compounds with suitable physical, chemical and biological properties.
6. Refers to a study subject who does not complete the protocol specified visits in a clinical trial.
7. Timelines for the submission of a summary report in case of premature termination/suspension of a clinical trial.
10. Refer to an individual's sense of general well-being and ability to perform various tasks.
11. Methods for the assessment and prevention of adverse events.
12. Title 21 of the CFR, Section 312 covers _________.

Down

2. Noxious and unintended response to medicinal product at any dose.
3. Early stages of a developing organism (from conception to 8th week of pregnancy).
4. Application filed to regulatory agencies for obtaining marketing authorization of a new drug.
5. An environment in which system access is controlled by persons, who are responsible for the content of electronic records.
8. Achievement of a desired outcome in a clinical trial.
9. Subsequent contact with a subject in order to assess current status of a subject's condition or outcome of an adverse event.

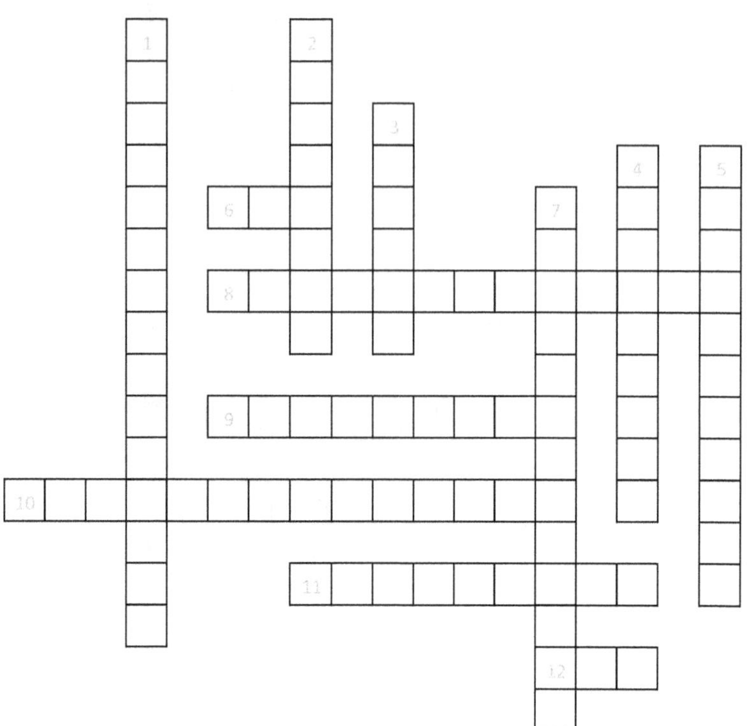

Across

6. Organization responsible for managing the investigator sites in a clinical trial.
8. Investigation of an approved drug in a new/unapproved indication.
9. A step by step procedure for making a series of choice, among alternative decision to reach an outcome.
10. Operational techniques and activities undertaken within the quality assurance system to verify that the requirements for quality of the trial-related activities have been fulfilled.
11. A list of drugs and their dosages to be used in a particular health plan.
12. A person employed at a trial site for coordinating the conduct of the trial.

Down

1. Rate and extent of a drug reaching the systemic circulation.
2. An event or outcome to answer the primary hypothesis of a clinical trial.
3. Clinical pharmacology studies in healthy volunteers (sometimes subjects), to determine the safety, tolerability, other dynamic effects of the drug/product, and its pharmacokinetic profile.
4. Non compliance to either protocol schedule of events or standard operating procedures.
5. The act of transforming document, text or phrases from one language to another.
7. Deviation from the protocol, standard operating procedures or applicable regulatory guidelines.

Crossword # 18

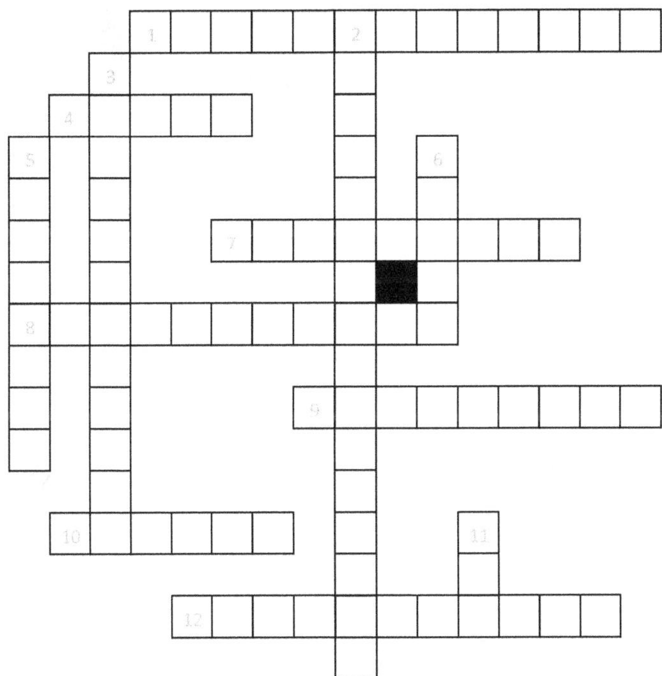

Across

1. Closing a clinical study after the same has been completed or prematurely terminated/suspended.
4. Regulatory body headed by DCGI.
7. A strategy employed in clinical trials comparing two treatments, where each patient receives both the treatments, one followed by other.
8. Refers to the degree to which the results of studies included in a systematic review are similar.
9. Enteric coating is done to achieve the dissolution of a drug in ____________.
10. Down coding or down grading is part of ____________ audit.
12. Articles published in peer-reviewed scientific journals.

Down

2. A method of providing experimental drugs/therapeutics, prior to their final regulatory approval for use in humans.
3. Med watch form for reporting safety information and adverse events to US-FDA .
5. A type of statistical chart that displays the distribution of levels of a categorical variable.
6. A person authorized to act on behalf of another person.
11. A classification of regulatory inspection outcome that requires voluntary action or response.

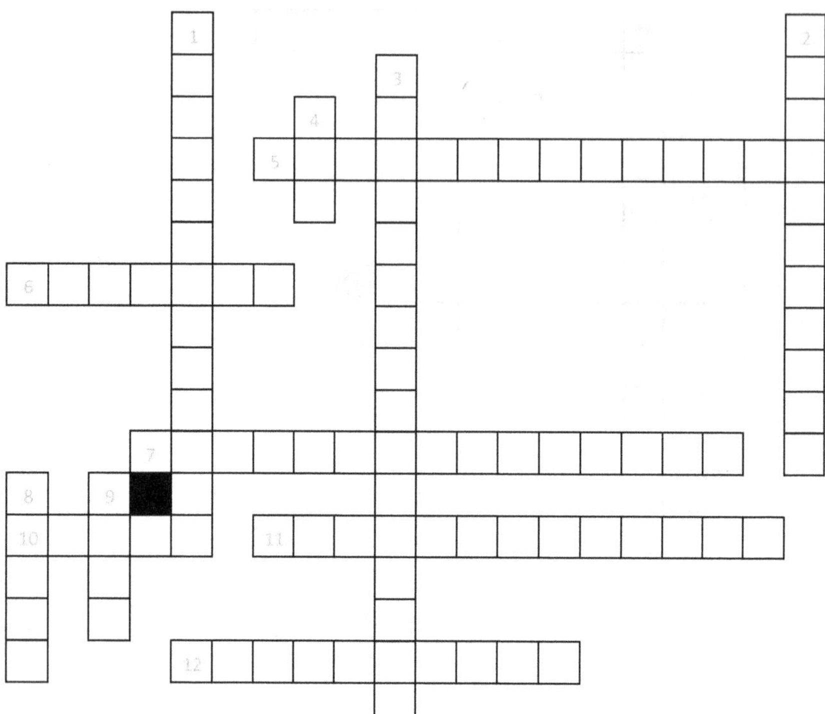

Across

5. Medical management of a patient based on established regimen or guidelines.
6. Controlled trials to evaluate safety and efficacy for determining a dose range to be studied in Phase-3 trials.
7. Total surface area of the human body which is widely used for the calculation of drug dosages of cancer medicines.
10. The difference between the smallest and largest values of a set of measurements.
11. Statistical principle which states that all randomized patients should be included for analysis.
12. United States agreement to cover all federal sponsored research by a common set of regulations.

Down

1. The code of medical ethics, designed to protect the safety and integrity of study participants and which came as a result of medical experimentation conducted by Nazis during World war II.
2. Actual cost associated with an activity.
3. A screening test to identify if a person has an inherited predisposition to a certain phenotype, or is at risk of producing offspring with inherited diseases or disorders.
4. A notification under ________________ scheme is required for all clinical investigation use of a product in Australia.
8. Any departure of the result from the "true" value is termed as________________
9. Application filed to seek approval for marketing a generic drug product.

Crossword # 20

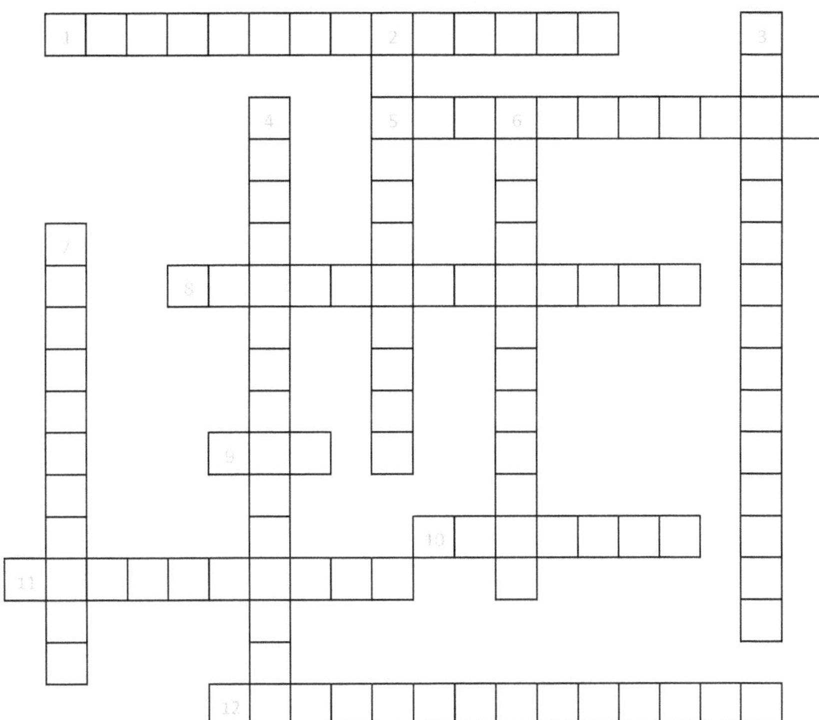

Across

1. The category of drugs that undergo parallel track review by FDA.
5. A mixture of chemicals and/or biological substances and excipients for preparing a dosage form.
8. Refers to records that describe or document study methods, conduct and results.
9. Practices required to be followed for the manufactured, handling and storage of Investigational Product.
10. The number assigned to an essential document in use.
11. An initial study to explore a new hypothesis.
12. A treatment designed to facilitate the process of recovery from injury, illness or disease to as normal a condition as possible.

Down

2. The unauthorized use of a drug for an indication, which is not approved by the regulatory authorities.
3. Studies conducted to estimate the rate and extent of drug absorption.
4. An independent body constituted of medical professionals and non medical members whose responsibility is to ensure the protection of the rights, safety and well being of human subjects.
6. Safety narratives prepared from serious adverse events.
7. A quality control process of standardizing the equipment, machines, apparatus to be used in scientific testing.

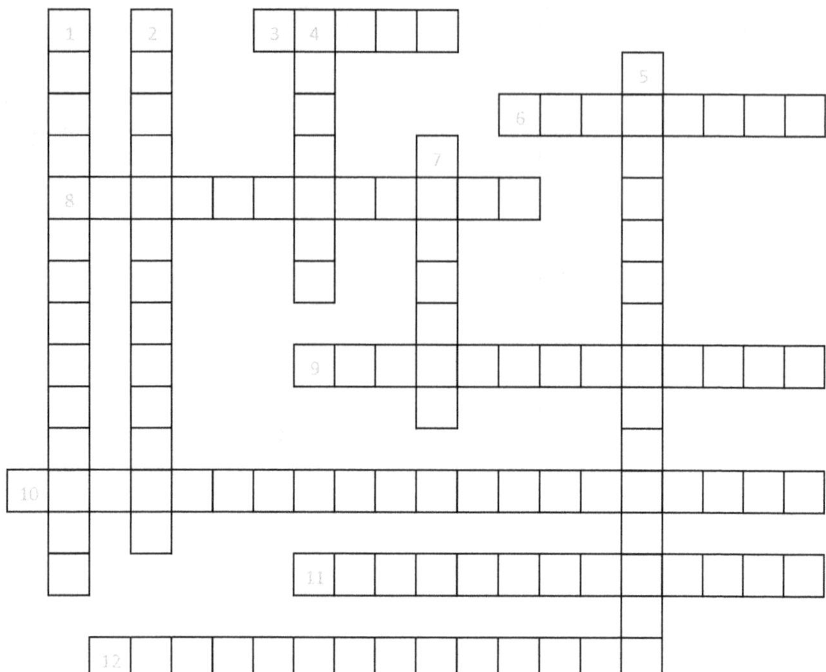

Across

3. The physical abnormalities that are linked to an adverse event.
6. Process of converting the data entered in an electronic data entry system to 'read only' format.
8. The decision of regulatory authorities to put a clinical study on hold.
9. A subject matter expert in a peer-group.
10. A compilation of the clinical and non clinical data on the investigational product(s).
11. Refer to an article that has a potential to become a successful drug through systematic clinical trial investigations.
12. Collection of information about each subject during the course of a trial.

Down

1. An authorization to undertake medical practice as per applicable regulations.
2. A comparison of case report form and ancillary data to the raw data in the clinical trial reporting database for the purpose of demonstrating the accuracy of data processing.
4. A device that is placed permanently into a tissue or surgically formed cavity of the human body.
5. A drug development approach that involves choosing a disease or biological target (such as enzyme, receptor, ion channel etc) to treat and then developing a model for that disease.
7. A process by which a subject voluntarily confirms his or her willingness to participate in a particular trial, after having been informed of all the aspects of the trial.

Crossword # 22

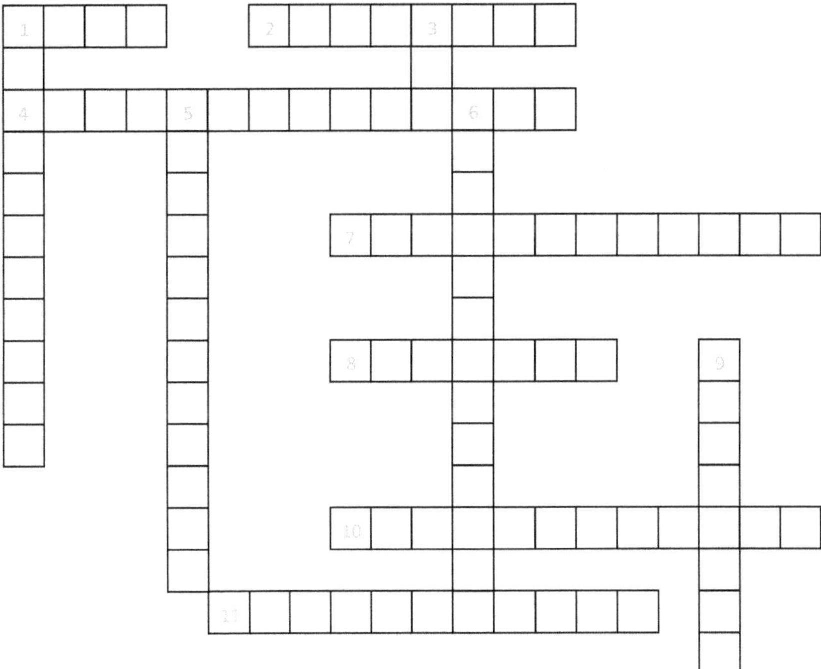

Across

1. The year in which Declaration of Helsinki was last amended.
2. Systematic investigation designed to develop new/innovative products, processes or services as well as improvisation of the existing products, processes or services.
4. A process of providing the health care services to an individual.
7. A person who is responsible for the conduct of a clinical trial at a site.
8. Concentration/strength of a drug, at which it is effective.
10. Refer to organisms of different but related species.
11. A contract to perform a part of or all the obligations of another contract.

Down

1. US-FDA regulations on protection of human subjects.
3. Refers to a treatment group in a randomized trial.
5. Combining the results of several studies that address a set of related research hypothesis.
6. Refers to an event or outcome to answer the primary hypothesis of a clinical trial.
9. A chemical synthesized or prepared from natural sources that is evaluated for its biological activities in preclinical tests.

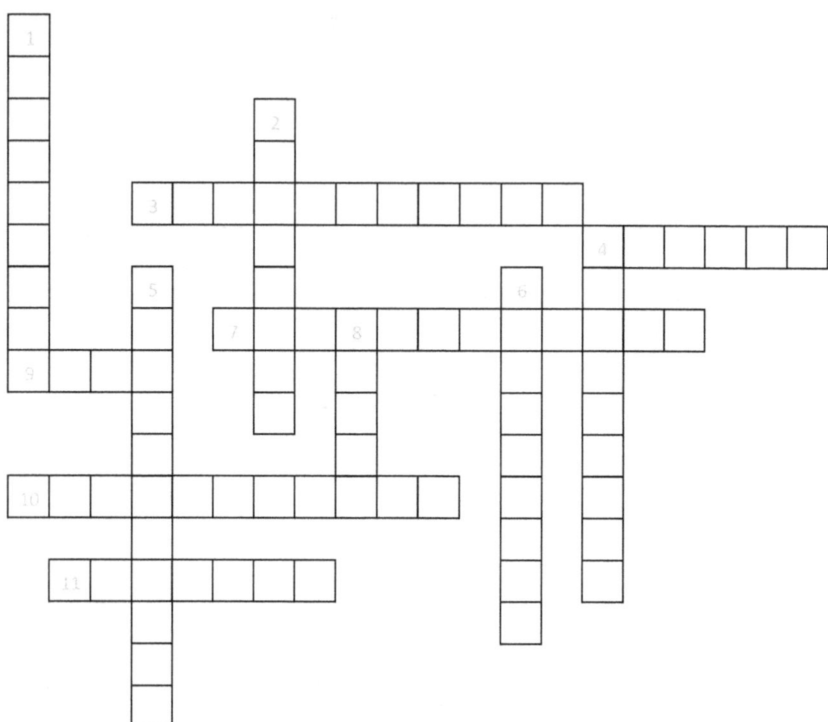

Across

3. The extent of relation between occurrence of an adverse event and administration of a drug/placebo.
4. A group of individuals identified on the basis of a common experience or characteristics that are usually monitored over time.
7. Compounds obtained from High Thoroughput Screening process that demonstrates the ability to interact with the desired target.
9. An independent data monitoring committee established by the sponsor to periodically assess the progress of a clinical trial, the safety data, and the critical efficacy endpoints.
10. Refers to the testing of experimental drugs in the test tube or in animals before trials in humans can be carried out.
11. The result of an activity, process, investigation or intervention.

Down

1. A statistical approach in which patients are analyzed according to the treatment that they received, rather than the one to which they were randomized.
2. An individual who is legally authorized to consent on behalf of a child, for participation in a clinical trial.
4. Term used for a potential drug substance.
5. Recording and reporting of false data or results.
6. Causative factor for a deviation or event.
8. An organization responsible to develop and support global platform-independent data standards that enable information system interoperability to improve medical research and related areas of healthcare.

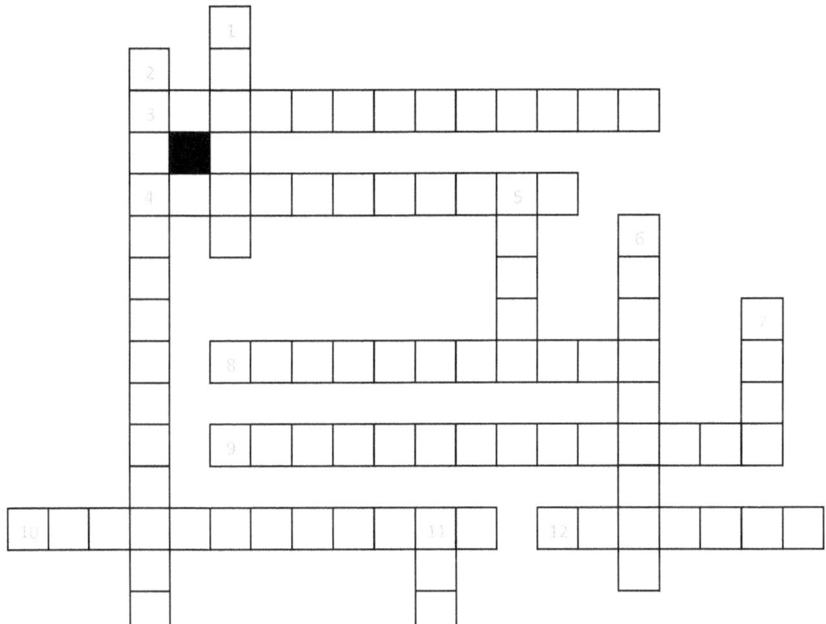

Across

3. Permission to use and share a subject's protected health information for the purpose of a research study.
4. Sign, symptom or laboratory results, not characteristic of normal individuals.
8. _______ _________Analysis is done to quantify the benefits associated with the use of a particular medication vis-à-vis direct cost implications.
9. Refer to facility, equipments, personnel and processes required to carry out a clinical trial.
10. A person legally competent to take decision about a subject's medical care.
12. The responsibility for the creation of essential trial documents like Protocol, ICF, and IB etc lies with________.

Down

1. A document that grants the sole right of an invention to its inventor.
2. A process of ensuring the accuracy and completeness of a clinical trial data using manual checks, computerized edits, reports or listing.
5. Time frame for submitting summary report to licensing authority (DCGI) for studies discontinued prematurely_________months.
6. The period of time during which a woman is providing her breast milk to an infant or child.
7. Most frequently occurring value in a set of data.
11. Guidelines for the choice of control group and related issue in clinical trials.

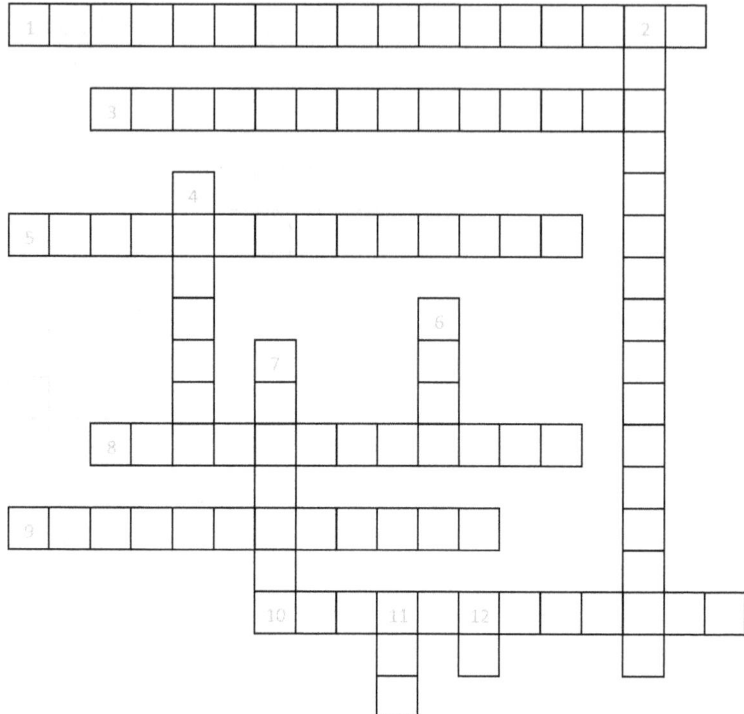

Across

1. Study of cost-benefit ratio of drugs with other therapies or with similar drugs.
3. A plan laid to define the monitoring visit intervals, source data verification requirements, protocol specifying monitoring instructions (if any) and other elements.
5. The process, documents and records to demonstrate that IP have been used in compliance with protocol.
8. Treatment of cancer using chemical agents.
9. A single legal entity that uses or discloses protected health information only for a part of its business operation.
10. Display of relation between two numeric variables while distinguishing between levels of categorical variables.

Down

2. A specific circumstance when the use of certain treatments could be harmful.
4. The principle of moral rightness in action or attitude.
6. A comparison of case report form and ancillary data to the raw data in the clinical trial reporting database for the purpose of demonstrating the accuracy of data process.
7. Deviation from standard operating procedure(s) or the regulatory guidelines is termed as ___________ deviation.
11. Regulatory agency in Australia.
12. Guidelines on general consideration for clinical trials.

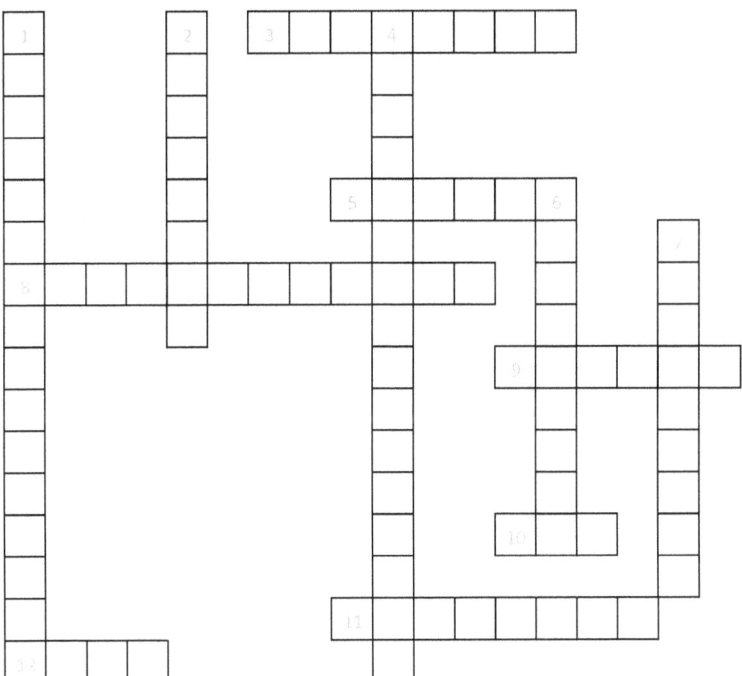

Across

3. FDA code that represents priority review for drugs having significant advantage over existing treatments.
5. Process of making a copy of important data, onto a different storage medium.
8. Primary object of a clinical trial (e.g. Drug, vaccine, behavior, device or procedure)
9. A computer that acts as a gateway for providing one or more services over a computer network.
10. Person who provides technical and statistical programming related expertise and advice.
11. Testing in human beings is known as _________ testing.
12. The main purpose of Phase-1 studies is to establish a ______ dosage range.

Down

1. A person who is independent of a trial, and who witness the adequacy of informed consent process, if the subject and his/her legally acceptable representative are unable to read and write.
2. The treatment group of a clinical trial.
4. Trials conducted to document both, therapeutic efficacy and tolerability between the generic and the original products.
6. ____________ health information refers to any information about health status, provision of health care or payment for health care that can be linked to an individual.
7. A condition of being confined to home and requiring considerable efforts and assistance to leave the home.

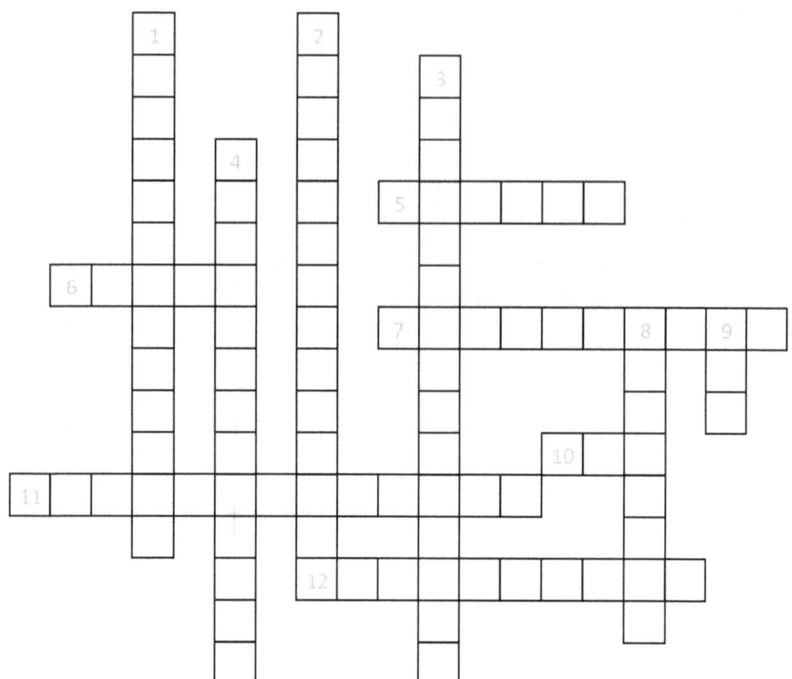

Across

5. The absence of extraneous material in a drug product.
6. Later stages of a developing organism (from conception to delivery).
7. The act of breaking the blinding codes of a clinical trial.
10. An independent entity, contracted by the sponsor to conduct drug development services on its behalf.
11. A reference book that contains official listing of marketed drugs.
12. Statistical analysis is a part of clinical data ___________ process.

Down

1. Three basic ethical principles: respect for persons, beneficence and justice.
2. Refers to pre-designed forms for recording trial data directly in to an electronic system.
3. Therapy provided to the patient in order to prevent the disease recurrence after the primary therapy has shown complete response.
4. A person (18 years of age and above), who is related and has maintained a regular contact with the prospective trial subject.
8. Procedure for breaking the treatment codes in a blinded clinical trial.
9. The paper used in Case Report Form (CRF) for manual entry.

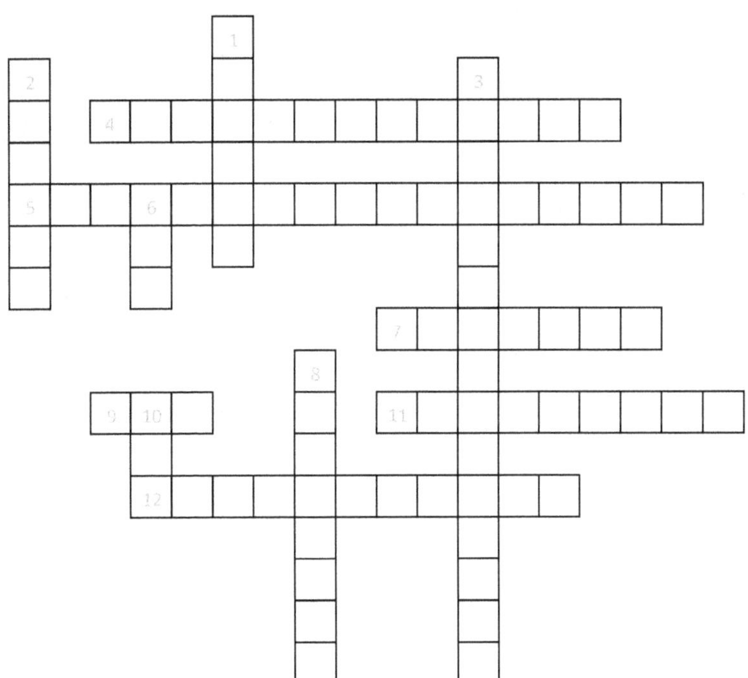

Across

4. Assays for the quantitative measurement of a drug, metabolites or chemicals in biological fluids.
5. Refers to a chemical molecule that after undergoing clinical trials could translate into a potential drug for the cure/treatment of a disease.
7. A report issued by FDA, following an audit that details the deficiencies requiring correction and other pertinent observations of the auditors.
9. The Periodic Safety Update Report should be submitted every ____ months for first two years, after approval of drug is granted to the applicant.
11. A name, word, symbol or phrase used to identify a particular product.
12. Accelerated approval is also known as accelerated ___________.

Down

1. Human micro dosing studies, designed to speed up the development of promising molecular entities or imaging agents.
2. A list of topics to be discussed in a meeting.
3. Adverse event in which a subject is at immediate risk of dying.
6. A person employed by a sponsor/CRO to monitor the conduct and progress of a trial.
8. A process to ascertain that management of clinical trial(s) and associated processes, utilize qualified individuals is referred to as ________ Qualification Review.
10. Application filed to regulatory agencies for initiating phase I trial .

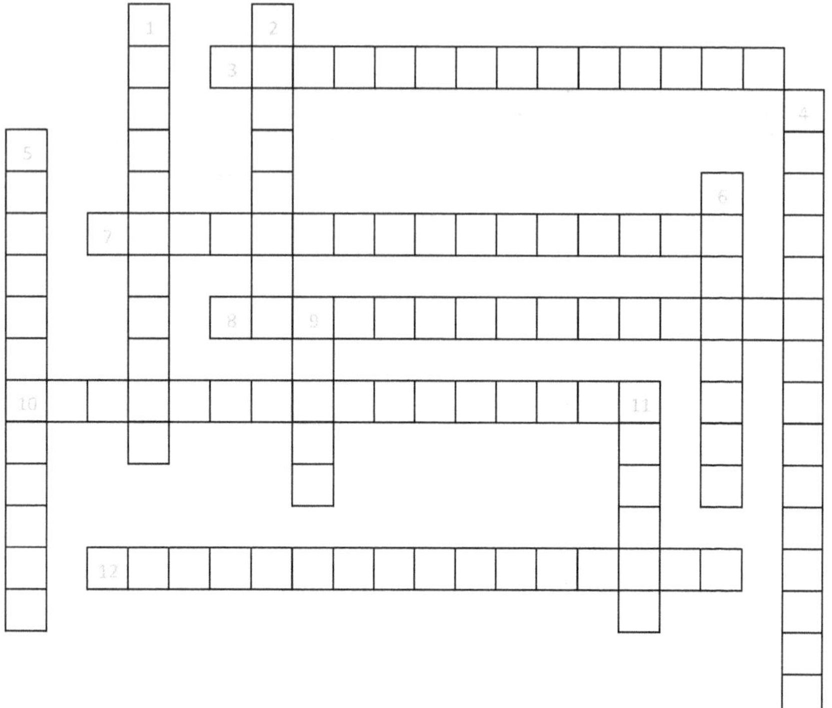

Across

3. Original documents, data and records.
7. Planned and systematic actions that are established to ensure that the trial is performed and the data are generated, documented and reported in compliance with GCP and applicable regulatory requirements.
8. A process by which subject voluntarily confirms his or her willingness to participate in a clinical trial.
10. A measure of how a subject, feels, functions or survives.
12. A person who is independent of the trial and who witnesses the adequacy of the informed consent process if the subject and/or his/her legally acceptable representative is illiterate.

Down

1. A type of bias that occurs when the two treatment groups that are being compared, contains different type of patients.
2. Unacceptable subject recruitment involving undue inducements, duress or indirect pressure to participate in a clinical trial.
4. A type of non-commercial Investigational New Drug Application submitted by a physician who both initiates and conducts an investigation and under whose immediate direction the investigational drug is administered or dispensed.
5. Storage of data under proper environment and access control, after the completion of a trial.
6. Intensity of an adverse event.
9. One of the aims of GLP is to help reduce the incidence of ____positive results.
11. Convenient and commonest drug dosage form.

Crossword # 30

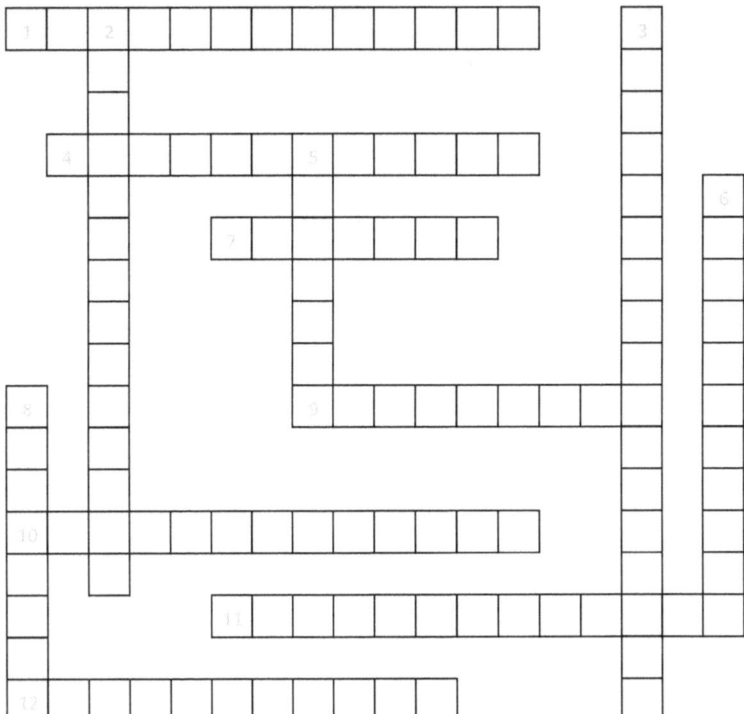

Across

1. Application filed primarily by companies, whose ultimate goal is to obtain marketing approval for the new product.
4. An environment in which the access to trial related information is not controlled.
7. Pilot clinical trials to evaluate safety in selected patient populations.
9. Refers to a state of being fair, so that the benefits and burdens of research are fairly distributed.
10. Necessity of informed consent was first described in ____________.
11. The process of assigning trial subjects to treatment group using an element of chance.
12. A medicinal product with the same active ingredient as that of an innovator drug.

Down

2. The information on overall general health, past illnesses and current medical problems of a subject.
3. Indicator of the relative variability of a variable around its mean.
5. A component or a substance that is analyzed employing an analytical technique.
6. Any public or private entity or medical or dental facility where clinical trials are conducted.
8. Clinical study design in which one or more parties to the trial are kept unaware of the treatment assignment(s).

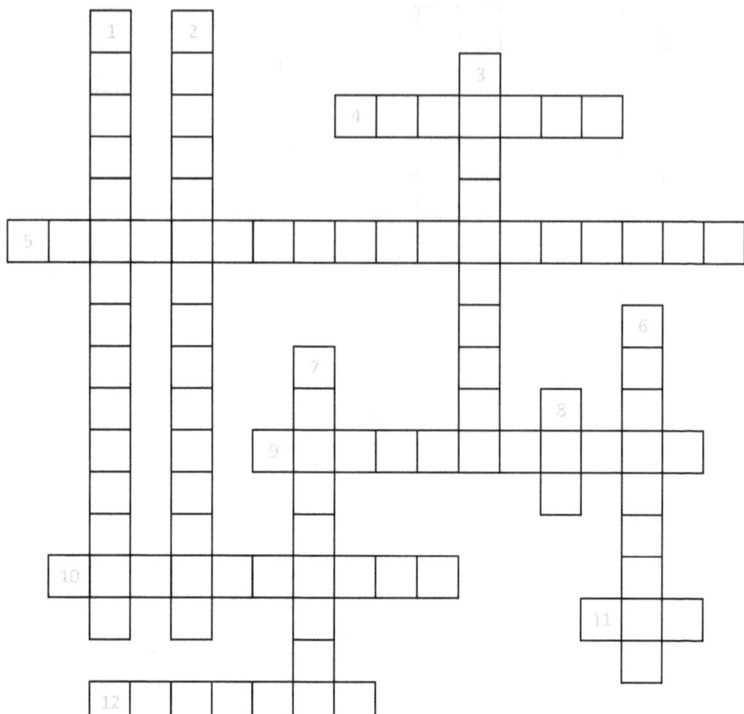

Across

4. A condition that impairs the normal functioning of an organism or body.
5. A non- interventional study, where investigator observes the subject and interprets the outcomes.
9. A process of estimating the magnitude of some attributes of an object such as its length or weight.
10. A government order with the force of the law.
11. An ICH defined format for regulatory submission that is considered acceptable in Japan, Europe, US and Canada.
12. The body of a deceased person used for imparting medical education.

Down

1. Advertisement for recruitment of study subjects require approval from ________
2. A group of trial participants having similar characteristics.
3. The native language of a country or a place is known as ______________ Language
6. De-identified information of a trial participant that in no way can disclose his/her identity.
7. Refers to any observable characteristic or trait of an organism such as morphology, biochemical or physiological properties.
8. A standard governing the manufacture of human and animal drugs and biologics intended to assure the quality and integrity of manufacturing data submitted to regulatory authorities.

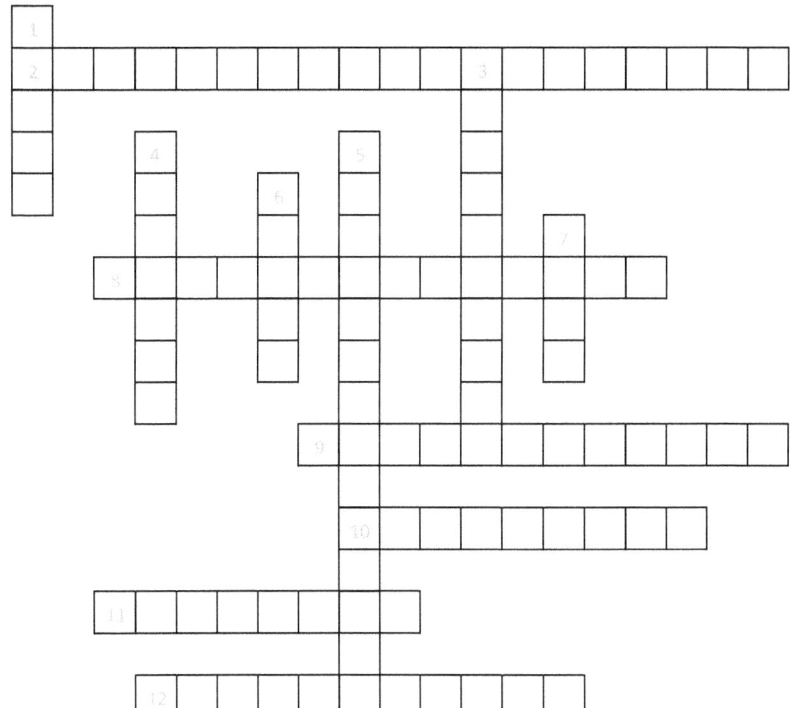

Across

2. Document that provides public assurance for the protection of rights, safety and wellbeing of human subjects involved in a clinical trial.
8. The process whereby one determines the clinical meaning or significance of data, after the relevant statistical analysis have been performed.
9. Data on important co-factors associated with a disease state.
10. A query generated during the data entry or review of a clinical trial data.
11. Federal Food and Drug Act in 1906 brought truth in ___________.
12. The design of a study in which neither the investigator nor the subject knows which medication the subject is receiving.

Down

1. Refers to an individual who has not attained the legal age of consenting to a trial, as per the applicable regulations.
3. An analysis involving a random variable.
4. Stakeholder responsible for the supervision, coordination and execution of successful data management of a clinical trial.
5. Documents narrating the conversation or discussion between two or more parties.
6. Number of years for which IRB/IEC should retain all records after the completion of the trial.
7. A factor, element, or course of action involving an uncertain, potentially negative outcome.

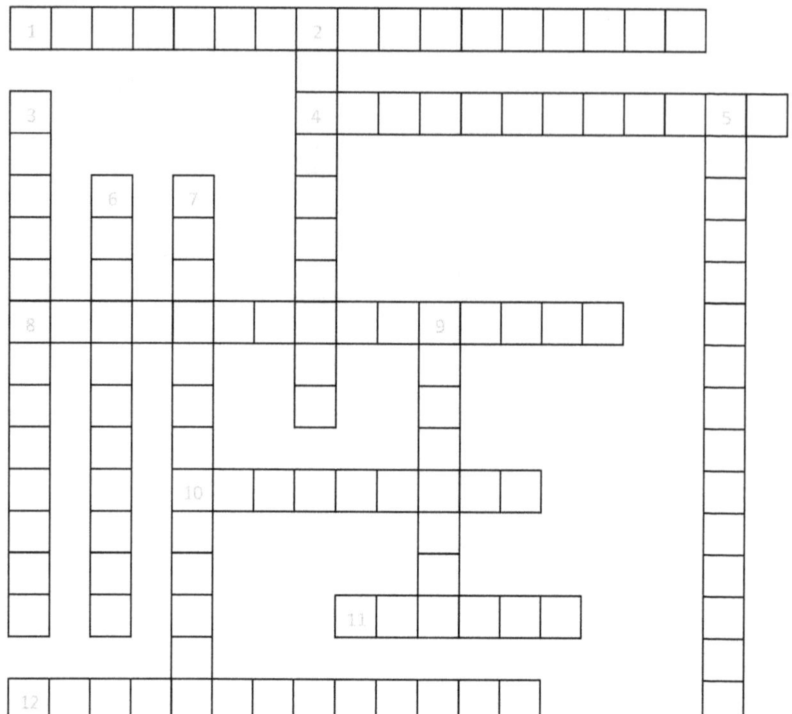

Across

1. Toxicological testing (up to 9 months) in two species of animals to determine the effect of drug on fertility and reproduction.
4. Analysis that combines the results of several studies to address a set of related research hypotheses.
8. A reference document that contains operating instructions for an equipment, activity or process.
10. Refers to the waivers that are provided under special circumstances with appropriate documentation of authorization.
11. Written instructions or rules to achieve uniformity, consistency and decision making.
12. Primary or secondary outcomes used to judge the effectiveness of a treatment.

Down

2. Adherence to study protocol, GCP guidelines and the applicable regulatory requirements.
3. Refers to the variability or differences between the results of studies included in a systemic review.
5. A pharmaceutical form of an active ingredient or placebo being tested or used as a reference in a clinical trial including a marketed product when used in an unapproved indication or dosage form is known as____Product
6. Complete records of patient's disease history entered in hospital files, out-patient charts or medical records.
7. The accuracy and validity of a given data.
9. Storage of data/records at the end of a trial for a stipulated timeframe.

Crossword # 34

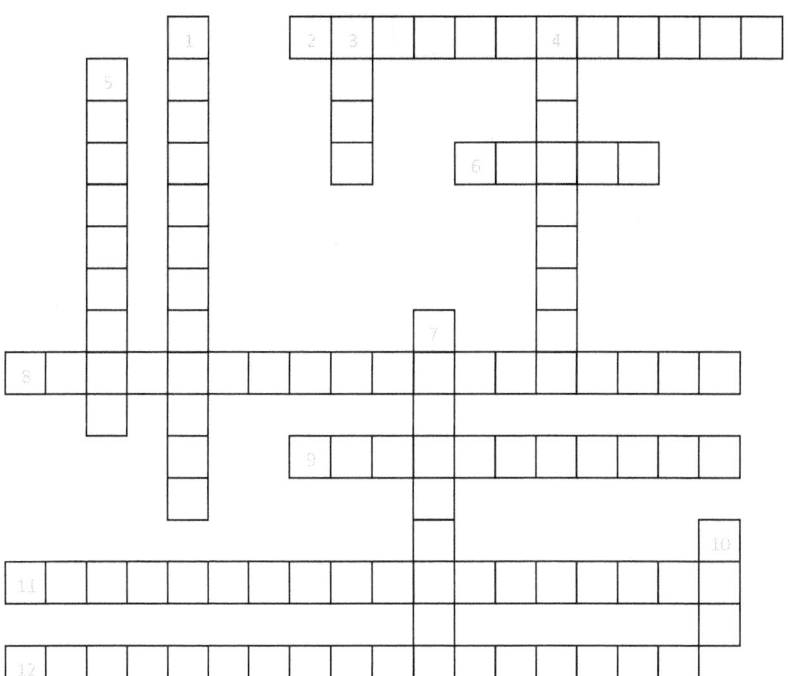

Across

2. US-FDA regulations on application for FDA approval to market a new drug.
6. Articles (other than food), intended for use in the diagnosis, cure, mitigation, treatment or prevention of disease in man or other animals.
8. The research in an institution that is supported by external funding.
9. Compounds obtained from High Throughput Screening Process.
11. Professional, personal or financial interest that can unduly bias an individual to perform his/her duties.
12. A laboratory finding which is taken as being predictive of important clinical outcomes in the patient.

Down

1. The allocation of specific trial related duties to the individual study team members at the investigator site is the responsibility of ____________.
3. The year in which ICH-Good Clinical Practice guidelines became effective.
4. A formal written, binding commitment.
5. The method by which the extent of relationship between a study drug and an adverse event is established: _________ assessment
7. The closeness with which results replicate analyses of a sample.
10. Drugs that are available for purchase without a physician's prescription.

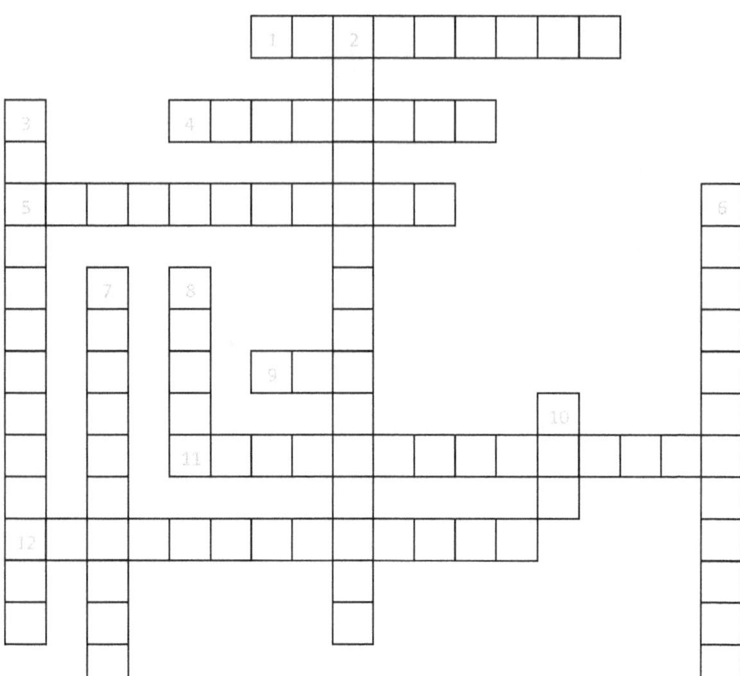

Across

1. Refer to intentionally misleading or withholding information.
4. Study of the physiological effects of drug on human body is called Pharmaco ______________.
5. Time period for which the patent of a drug is valid.
9. A person or an organization contracted by the sponsor to perform one or more of a sponsor's trial related duties and functions.
11. A tool used during the randomization process to ensure an exact balance between the treatment arms with respect to key patient factors that are strongly related to the outcome variable.
12. A scale for ranking items where the distance between adjacent points are equal.

Down

2. Statistical tests used for drawing conclusions about differences between two or more groups.
3. New Drug Application is filed to obtain marketing ______________.
6. Time frame for reporting SAEs to IRB/EC as per Schedule-Y.
7. Distribution free test that is applied when the data is not normally distributed is referred to as non ______________ test.
8. Aerosols are used to deliver the drug in __________.
10. A classification of regulatory inspection outcome that does not require any action or response.

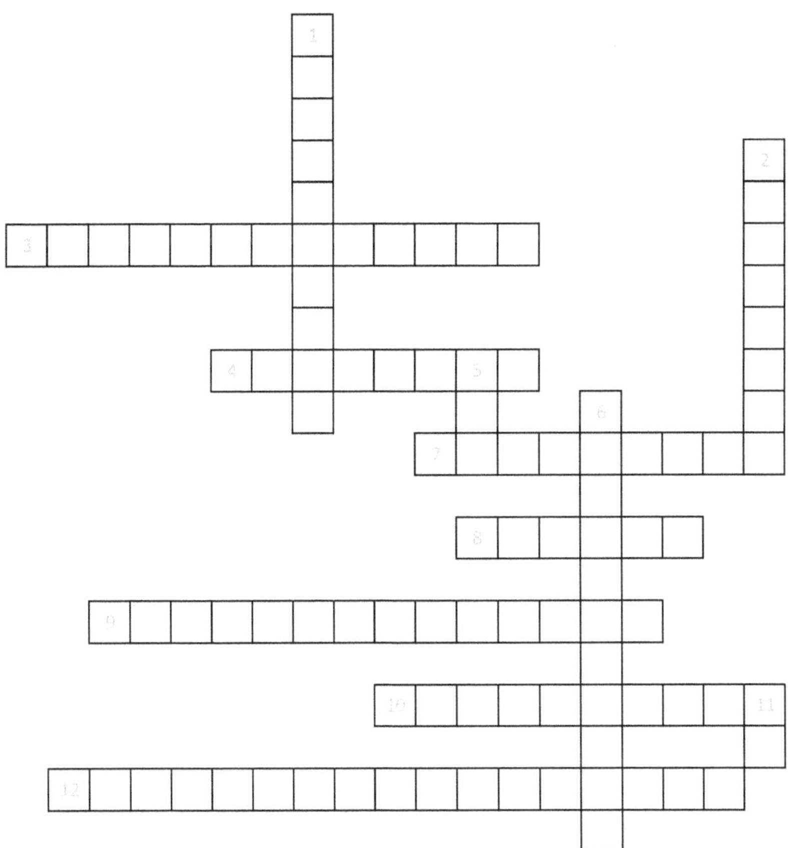

Across

3. A mechanism by which the access to clinical trial facility or documents is restricted to authorized individuals.
4. A written, dated and signed agreement between two or more involved parties that sets out arrangements on delegation and distribution of tasks and financial matters.
7. A particular method of performing a task.
8. Investigational New Drug Application is filed to initiate the testing of a drug in _____.
9. A document that lists the core job functions of a job.
10. Number of patients required to achieve the desired statistical significance in a clinical trial.
12. Relationship of significance in the life of a research subject such as parent-child, spousal, employer-employee.

Down

1. The act of overseeing the progress of a clinical trial.
2. An electronic platform that contains the data generated from a clinical trial.
5. Code of Federal Regulation is commonly denoted as _________.
6. Substances or agents that can interfere with normal embryonic development.
11. ICH consolidated Guideline on Good Clinical Practice (GCP).

Crossword # 37

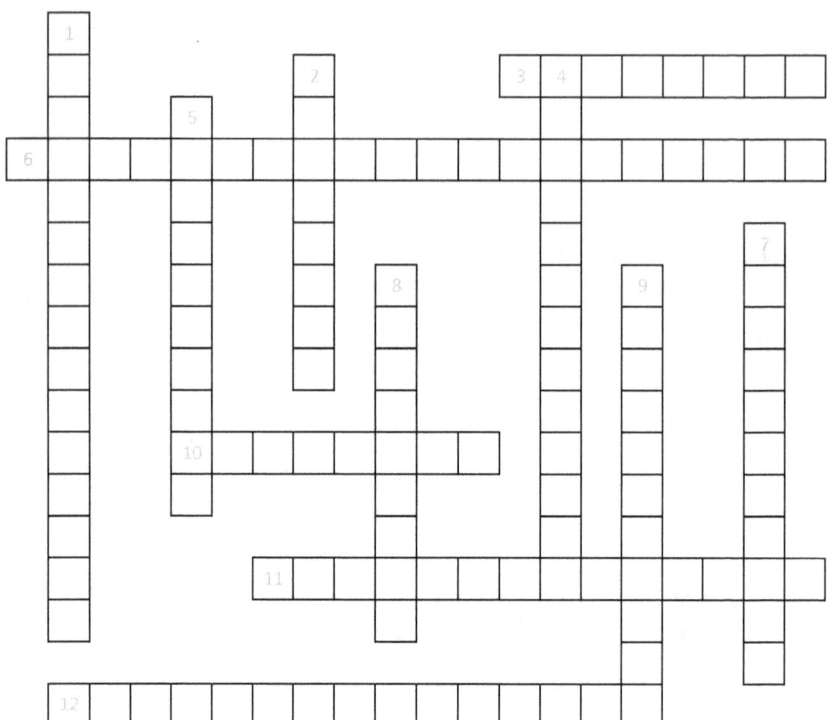

Across

3. Ethical guidelines for biomedical research onhuman subject.
6. Any untoward medical occurrence that at any dose results in death or hospitalization or disability or congenital anomaly or is life-threatening.
10. Number of Principles in ICH-GCP Guidelines.
11. The drug products that have the same active ingredient, dosage, form, route of administration, strength or concentration are as called ________equivalents.
12. Process by which vernacular language translation of a trial document is back translated in to english.

Down

1. A type of non-commercial IND.
2. A site visit by an FDA investigator to find out whether GCP requirements are being followed.
4. A clinical trial database in which all the validation queries have been resolved and which is ready for analysis.
5. A process by which compliance with essential requirements is evaluated (Assessment).
7. Ownership of sole rights of a document, process or product.
8. A document that contains results of the laboratory tests.
9. A measurement of the strength of the relationship between two variables.

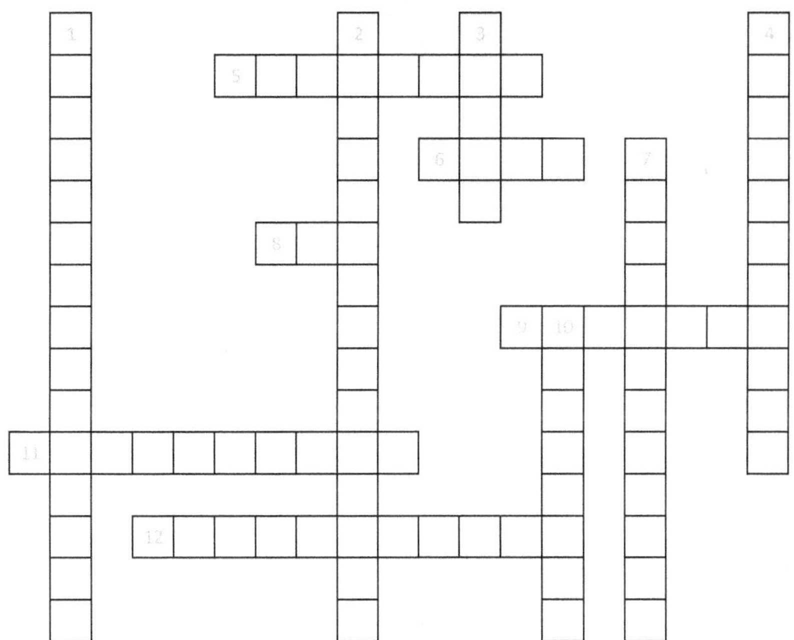

Across

5. A written, formal clarification in an essential trial document.
6. Recorded information regardless of form (manual or electronic).
8. Association responsible for developed Declaration of Helsinki.
9. Respect for person, beneficence, justice are the three principles discussed in the _________ Report.
11. Cognitive impairment refers to a medical condition in which an individual's capacity for judgment and reasoning is significantly ___________.
12. Quantitative data such as number of patients, number of visits etc.

Down

1. Official daily publication for rules, proposed rules and notices of federal agencies and organization in United States.
2. Technique involving genetic linkage studies and genetic association studies.
3. Suspected Unexpected Serious Adverse Reactions.
4. Publishing the results of a clinical trial in a peer-reviewed journal.
7. The study of the effect of drugs on living organisms.
10. A product's ability to produce beneficial effects for a disease.

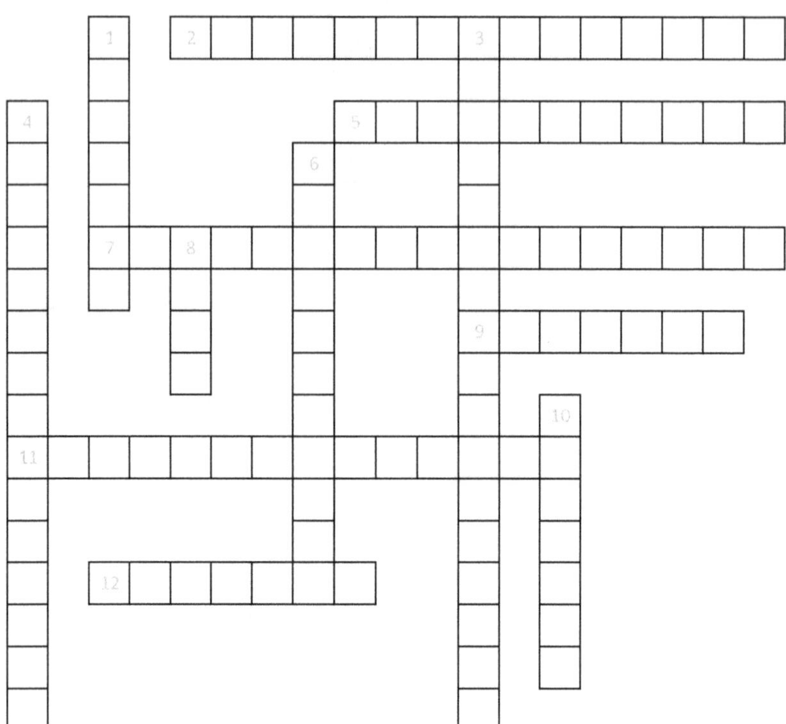

Across

2. Compassionate use IND is also known as ___________.
5. ____________ statement is signed by investigator(s) at the end of the trial to document their compliance with ICH-GCP and applicable regulatory requirements.
7. Criteria that makes a subject eligible for a clinical trial.
9. Official or legal permission to an individual or organization by a competent authority to engage in a practice, occupation or activity.
11. A file that contains all the essential trial documents at a trial site.
12. A process of submitting competitive proposals to a trial sponsor.

Down

1. Post marketing studies to collect the additional safety data from a larger patient population.
3. Investigator is responsible for obtaining the ERB/IEC approval of the trial at a ________.
4. Studies that determines the maximum tolerated dose.
6. ____________ certificate is a document that captures the description and the quantity of a clinical trial material destroyed.
8. Regulatory Authority that grants the permission for conducting clinical trials in Europe.
10. Refer to newborn baby.

Crossword # 40

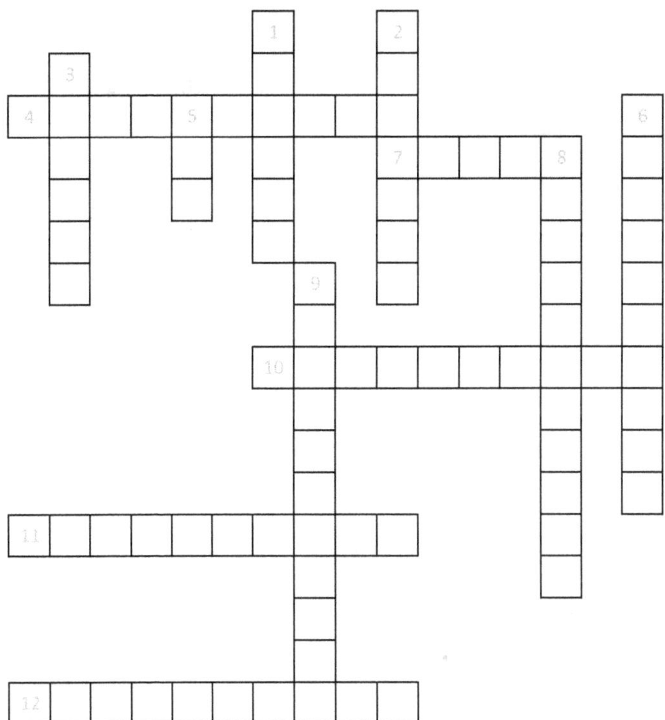

Across

4. All information in original record and certified copies of original records of clinical findings, observations or other activities in a clinical trial.
7. A document for identifying a drug/placebo in compliance with applicable regulations and appropriateness of the instructions provided to the subjects.
10. A systematic and independent examination of trial related activities and documents.
11. Time frame in which an IND becomes effective if the FDA does not disapprove it.
12. Text or numbers generated during the analysis of a clinical trial data.

Down

1. The process of assigning data to categories, having a unique identifier for analysis.
2. A pre-set standard for measuring the outcome.
3. Application for permission to conduct clinical trials for New Drug/IND in India is made in _________Format
5. A printed, optical or electronic document designed to record all of the protocol-required information on each trial subject.
6. Refers to a condition that forms the basis for the initiation of a treatment or of a diagnostic test.
8. Drugs that have immediate authorization and can be sold in a country.
9. A measure that determines the degree to which the movement of two variables is associated.:- ____________Coefficient

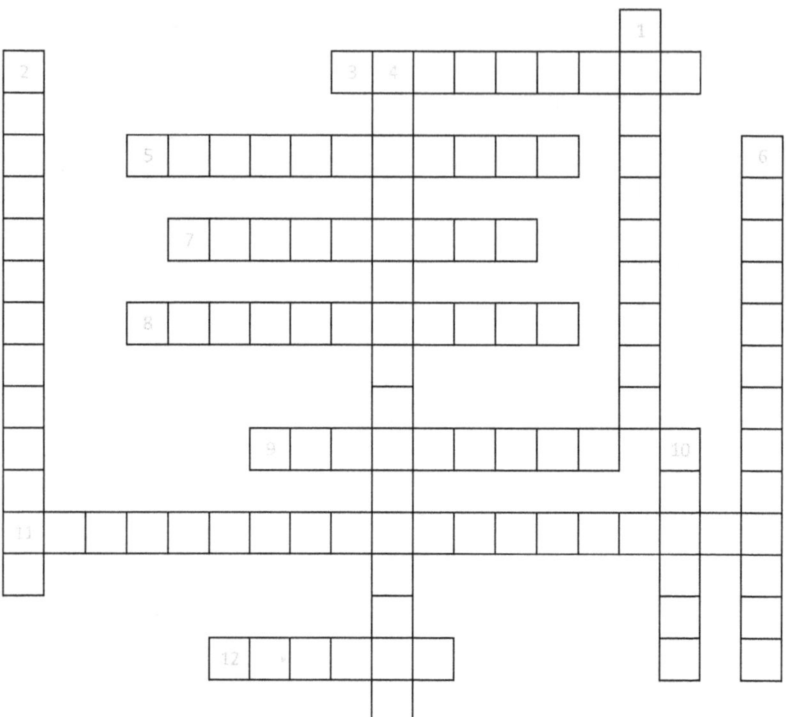

Across

3. Written description of a change(s) to protocol or formal clarification of a protocol is known as protocol _____________.
5. A clinical trial in which two or more doses of an agent are tested against each other to determine which dose works best and is least harmful_________________study.
7. A type of study in which both the investigator and subject knows which treatment the subject is receiving.
8. The extent of harm or discomfort anticipated from a clinical trial which is not greater than the routine practice.
9. Refers to a stage of being balanced or in equilibrium.
11. A physician whose practice is not limited to a specialty.
12. Therapeutic Exploratory Trials.

Down

1. An official review of documents, facility, records and any other resources related to clinical trial by a regulatory authority at the site of the trial.
2. Technique that uses living organisms, or substances from organism, biological systems, or processes to make or modify a product or process, to change plants or animals, or to develop micro-organisms for specific uses.
4. A state in which a person is not able to manage his/her affairs or to make a choice due to a psychiatric or developmental disorder.
6. A technique of modifying an existing compound chemically to act on a selected target______________chemistry.
10. An element of chance or having no specific pattern.

Crossword # 42

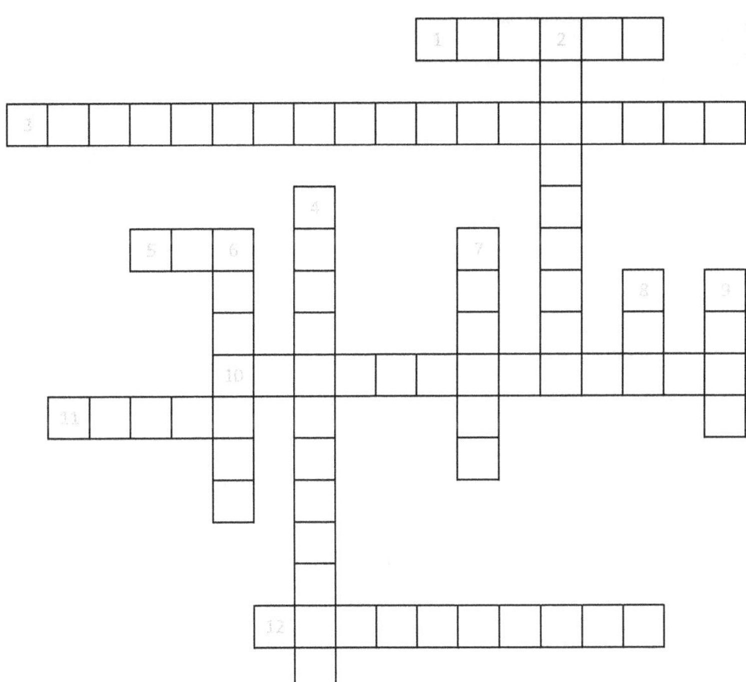

Across

1. A supplier of goods or services.
3. A non interventional study conducted according to routine medical practice.
5. A standard for the conduct and reporting of non-clinical laboratory studies intended to assure the quality and integrity of safety data submitted to regulatory authorities.
10. Data on the stability of a drug product under routine and accelerated stability conditions.
11. Storage area on a computer's hard drive where the web page and/or graphic elements are stored temporarily.
12. A list of relevant published literature on a topic along with complete citation.

Down

2. A new invention.
4. Yearly review of the progress of a trial by ethics committee(s) or regulatory agencies.
6. Trials conducted after regulatory submission but prior to the drug's approval or launch.
7. Conforming to an accepted standard of human behavior.
8. A document signed and dated by investigator and the sponsor of a trial, describing the responsibility, timelines, payment schedule and other relevant terms.
9. An arithmetic value that is obtained by summing up all the observations and dividing by the total number of observations.

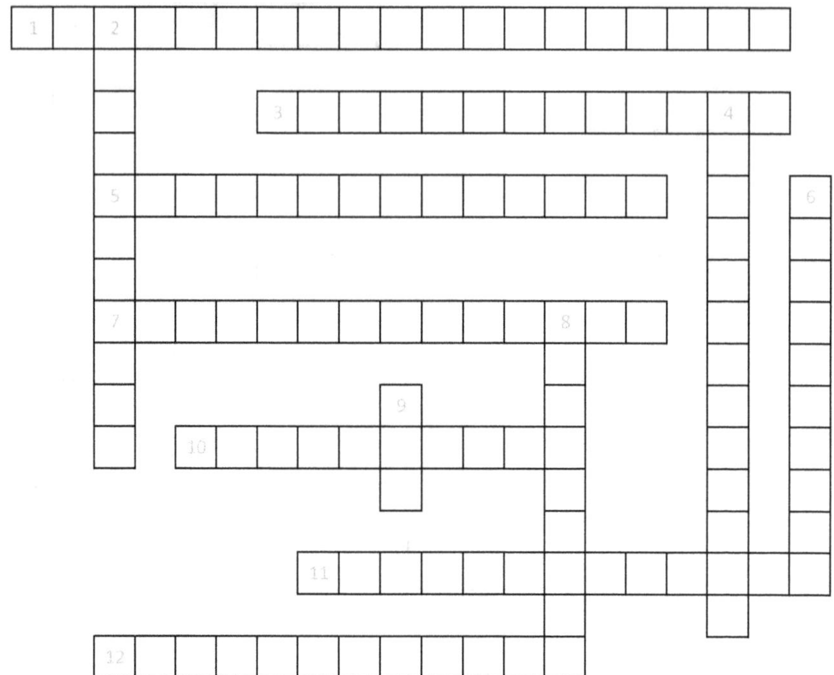

Across

1. The extent to which tests or procedures assess the same characteristic, skill or quality.
3. A list published on US FDA's website containing the names of personnel that have been disqualified from conducting clinical trials on grounds of medical fraud.
5. A patient who is no longer in touch with the site person/site during the trial.
7. A medically qualified personnel in an organization who supports the marketing and/ or research department.
10. A marketed product or placebo used as a reference in a clinical trial.
11. Non-skilled personal care such as help with activities of daily living like bathing, dressing, eating etc.
12. Toxicity studies for 18-24 months in vivo and in vitro are done to assess ____________.

Down

2. A unique identifier assigned to a clinical study for its easy identification.
4. Time frame for reporting fatal or life-threatening unexpected ADRs to regulatory agencies as per ICH-GCP (no later than) ____________ Days
6. Individuals whose willingness to volunteer in a clinical trial may be unduly influenced in case of his refusal to participate __________________ subjects.
8. The absence of viable, contaminating microorganisms.
9. Ancillary trial data is generally not collected on ____________.

Crossword # 44

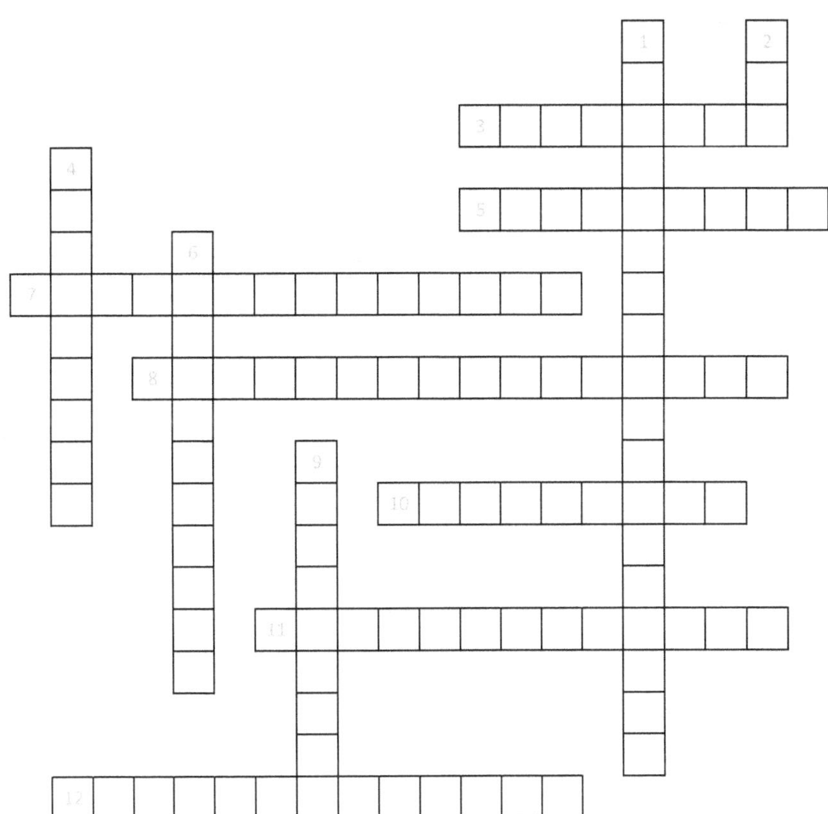

Across

3. Pharmaco____________ refers to the physiological effect of drug on human body.
5. Errors in either collection or recording of clinical trial data.
7. An Individual or juridical or other body authorized under applicable law to consent on behalf of a prospective subject for participation in a clinical trial.
8. A type of retrospective study comparing persons with a given condition and persons without the condition with respect to antecedent factors.
10. Refers to a factor that defines a system and its performance.
11. Drugs that are approved by a regulatory agency to be marketed in a country.
12. Primary or secondary outcome(s) used to judge the effectiveness of a treatment.

Down

1. Authority that grants trial permission and monitors compliance with applicable regulatory guidelines.
2. Studies conducted to assess the long term safety of the approved and marketed drug/ device.
4. Refer to the quantity of goods and materials available in the stock.
6. Needle placed in the arm with blood thinner to prevent the blood from clotting inside the needle or tubing.
9. Formal submission of a trial application by a sponsor to the regulatory agency, followed by obtaining no objection for initiating the trial is referred as Clinical Trial ____________.

Crossword # 45

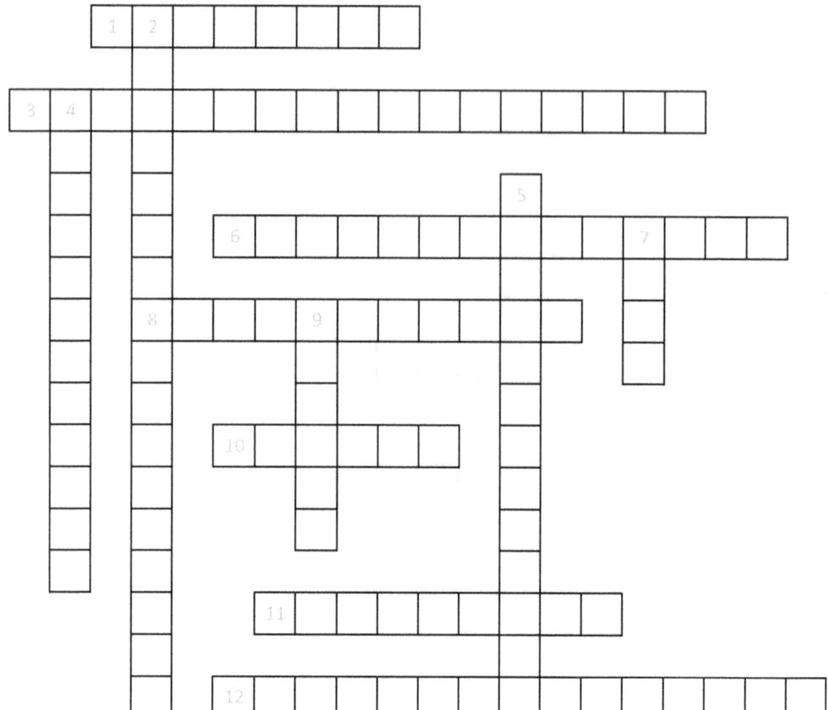

Across

1. An amendment in the existing documents or processes.
3. Use of available published data as a control arm.
6. US-FDA regulations on reporting of IND safety reports for drugs and biologics.
8. A designation of the US-FDA to indicate a therapy developed to treat a rare disease.
10. Sponsor-FDA meeting held to discuss the presentation of data (both paper and electronic) in support of the drug application.
11. The relation of an adverse event (effect) to the study drug/procedure.
12. Prevention of disclosure of proprietary information to unauthorized individuals.

Down

2. Extending the expiry date on the label of an investigational product.
4. Reporting of ongoing safety, progress reports, and re-approvals to IRB is the responsibility of ____________.
5. A drug discovery approach that involves finding a drug or group of drugs which works on the selected targets.
7. The year in which Declaration of Helsinki came in force.
9. A process by which a child voluntarily confirms his/her willingness to participate in a clinical trial.

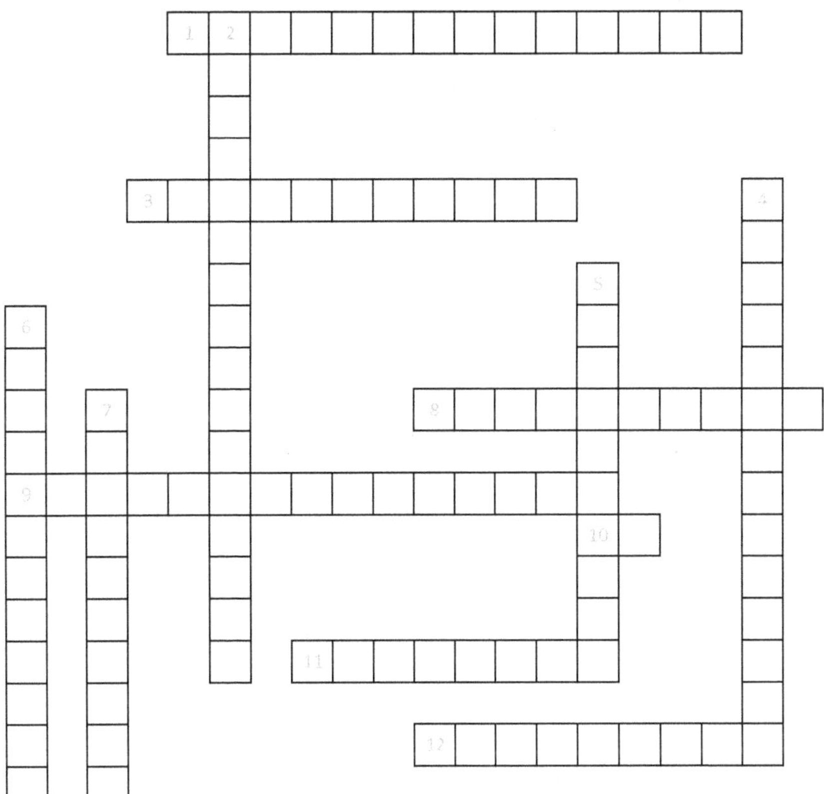

Across

1. Randomization scheme that changes over time depending on the data generated in a trial.
3. The notes to explain the deviation/ violation of a particular activity/ process.
8. A person with the authority to oversee the work of a person or group.
9. Target Selection is being revolutionized through the application of _____________.
10. A document containing the details on the qualification, experience and personal details of a person.
11. A product's ability to produce beneficial effect on the course or duration of a disease.
12. A state of physical and mental soundness.

Down

2. An electronic signature based upon cryptographic methods of originator authentication such that the identity of the signer and the integrity of the data can be verified.
4. The process of verifying the data entered in the case report form against the source data in order to establish its accuracy and completeness.
5. Characteristic of a drug used to determine crystal morphology and particle size.
6. The Science of drug and their clinical use is called clinical _______________.
7. The documentation of activities that allows reconstruction of the course of events.

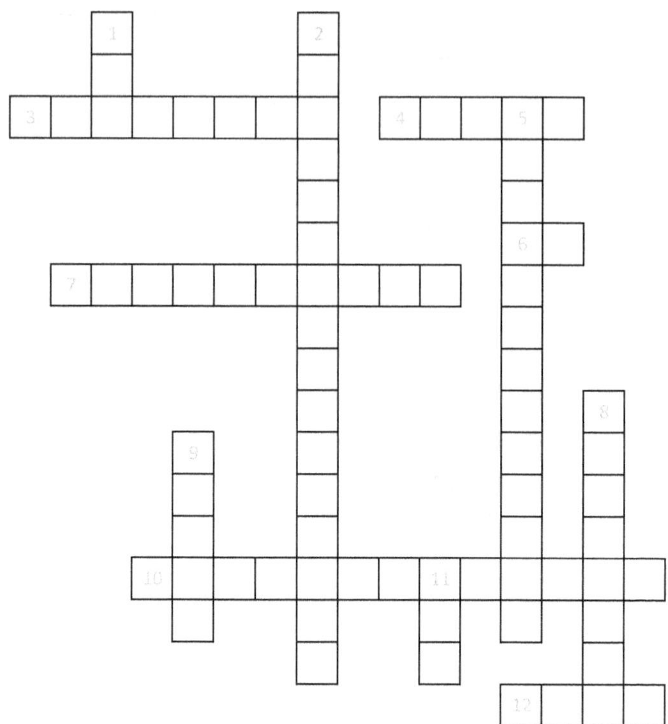

Across

3. A formal written agreement which sets forth the working arrangements, between two or more parties.
4. An act causing physical, social or mental harm or discomfort.
6. Guidelines for ethnic factor in the acceptability of foreign clinical data.
7. The act of overseeing the progress of a clinical trial, and of ensuring that it is conducted, recorded and reported in accordance with the protocol, standard operating procedure, GCP and applicable regulatory requirements.
10. Recording of false data or results and reporting them.
12. An automated interactive voice response system used to randomize or withdraw the patients in a clinical trial.

Down

1. Number of principles in Nuremberg Code.
2. Process of checking the accuracy of the data that has been entered into a computer database.
5. Report prepared from a serious and unexpected adverse experience.
8. A person who is confined to custody.
9. ANDA does not require incorporation of animal and ________ data to establish safety and efficacy.
11. An annual codification of the general and permanent rules published in the Federal Register (US), by the executive departments and agencies of the Federal Government.

Crossword # 48

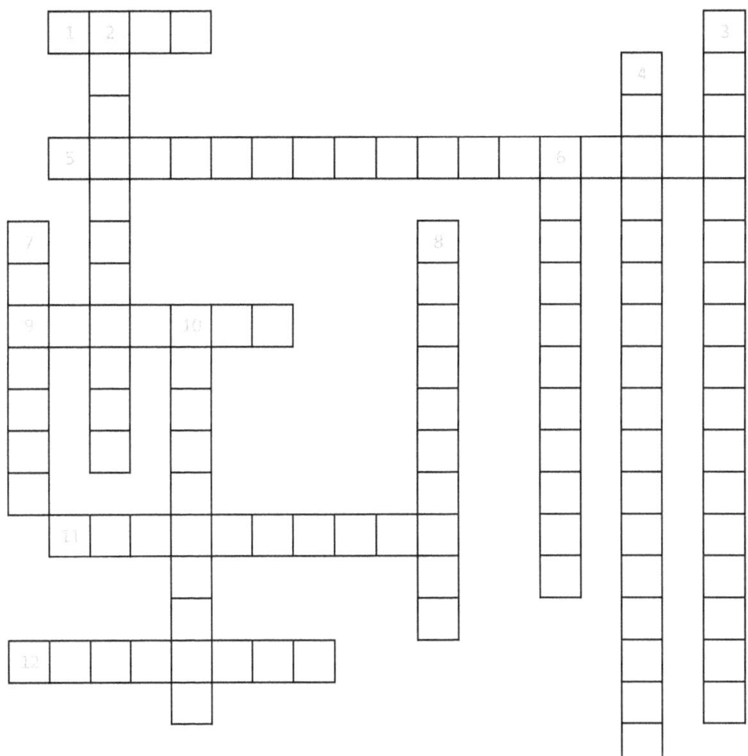

Across

1. Regulatory Authority responsible for regulating clinical trials in India.
5. A statistical test that provides an analysis of variance by ranks and is the non-parametric equivalent of the F-test for analysis of variance.
9. Dissection of a dead body to determine the cause of death and relevant medical facts.
11. Codes used by the FDA to classify medical devices according to the potential risks or hazards.
12. A written description of a work plan.

Down

2. A measure of the strength of the relationship between two variables.
3. Clinical trials conducted according to a single protocol at more than one site and by more than one investigator.
4. The concentration range over which a drug has a therapeutic effect, without having unacceptable toxicity.
6. Discovery by chance.
7. A list of commitments and requirements by the FDA for each investigator performing drug/biologic studies.
8. The scientific rationale behind a research project.
10. Form 44 represents __________ to conduct clinical trial in India.

Crossword # 49

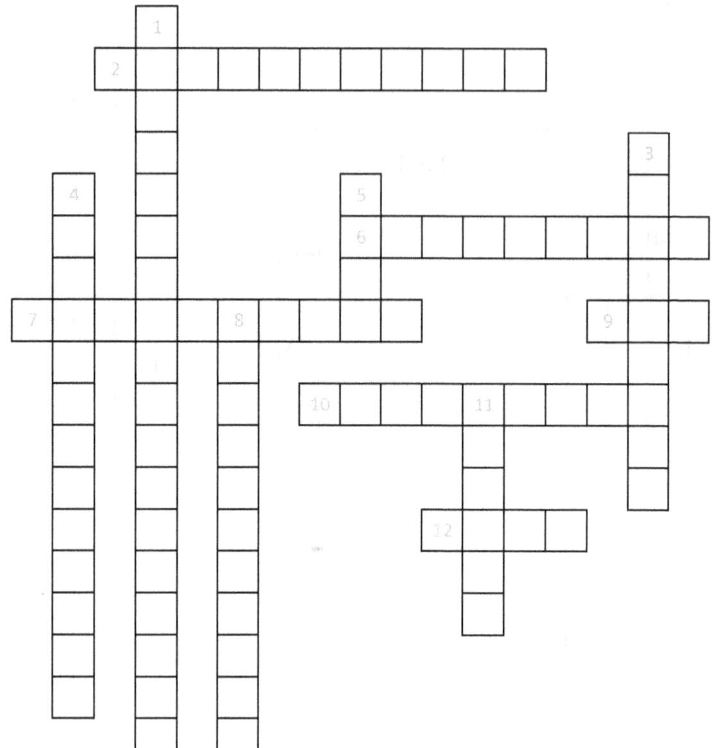

Across

2. Analytical reports/tables for a given dataset.
6. A trial design in which all the involved parties knows the treatment group to which a subject is assigned.
7. An objective or goal to be achieved in a stipulated time-frame.
9. A form signed by the investigator and sub-investigators, to disclose their financial interest in the sponsor company, for whom they intent to participate in a clinical trial.
10. Ethical principle of assigning patient to different arms, where the clinician does not have any preference for one arm over the others.
12. Safety reporting of marketed drugs in a specified period of time (generally on an annual basis).

Down

1. Refer to pre-treatment evaluations on study subjects as they enter a clinical trial.
3. Changes made to essential trial documents (such as protocol, ICD, IB etc.) that have an impact on overall conduct of the study.
4. Number of new events in a population during a specified period of time.
5. The amount of a drug to be used for a medical condition.
8. Written description of the outcome of a trial enumerating the clinical and statistical interpretations is known as Clinical __________.
11. Clinical investigation studies in subjects with the target disease, to determine efficacy, safety and tolerability in carefully controlled dose-ranging studies.

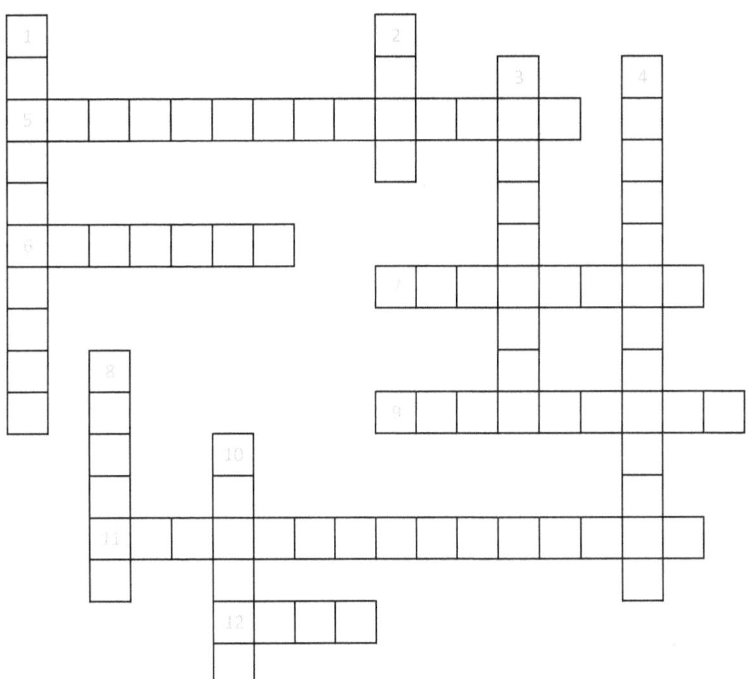

Across

5. The process of assessing the readiness of an investigator site for initiating the enrolment in a clinical trial.
6. Willful oversight in performing a particular activity.
7. An adverse effect produced by a drug that is detrimental to the participant's health.
9. A document that set forth the payment terms in a clinical trial is known as; Letter of_____________.
11. A type of non-commercial IND.
12. The year in which Nuremberg code was enforced.

Down

1. Personnel that have been assigned specific trial related duties.
2. A preconceived personal preference or inclination that might influence the assessment of the trial.
3. Refers to a variable that has an influence on another dependent variable.
4. A document used for subject recruitment after obtaining EC approval that contains non-coercive trial information.
8. Therapeutic Confirmatory Trials.
10. Permission to import the drug may be obtained by applying in _______ for a test license.

Crossword # 51

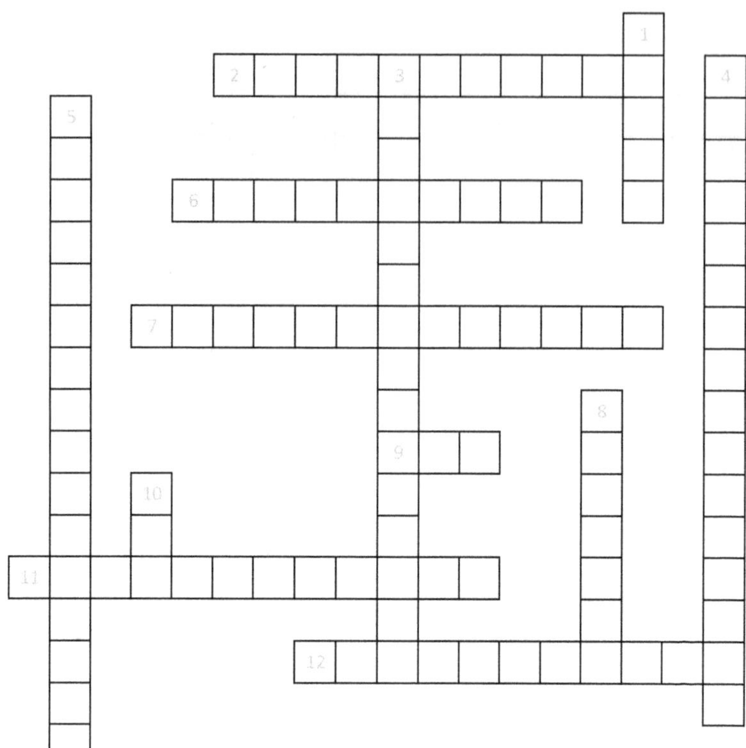

Across

2. A variable that is based on categorical data and cannot be measured numerically.
6. All information in original record and certified copies of original records of clinical findings, observations or other activities in a clinical trial.
7. An important factor in the absorption of a drug.
9. An individual who shares study responsibilities with the investigator at the site.
11. A type of non-commercial IND.
12. A medical procedure that doesn't involve skin break.

Down

1. A fatal outcome of an adverse event.
3. A legal statement or document indicating protection or exemption from liability for compensation of damages from a third party is known as _____________ letter.
4. A type of in vitro and in vivo toxicological testing for 18-24 months to determine the mutagenic potential of a drug.
5. Trials that are conducted to find better tests or procedures for diagnosing a particular disease or condition.
8. Timeframe for reporting SAEs to Sponsor.
10. Certificate of analysis is commonly denoted as _____________.

Crossword # 52

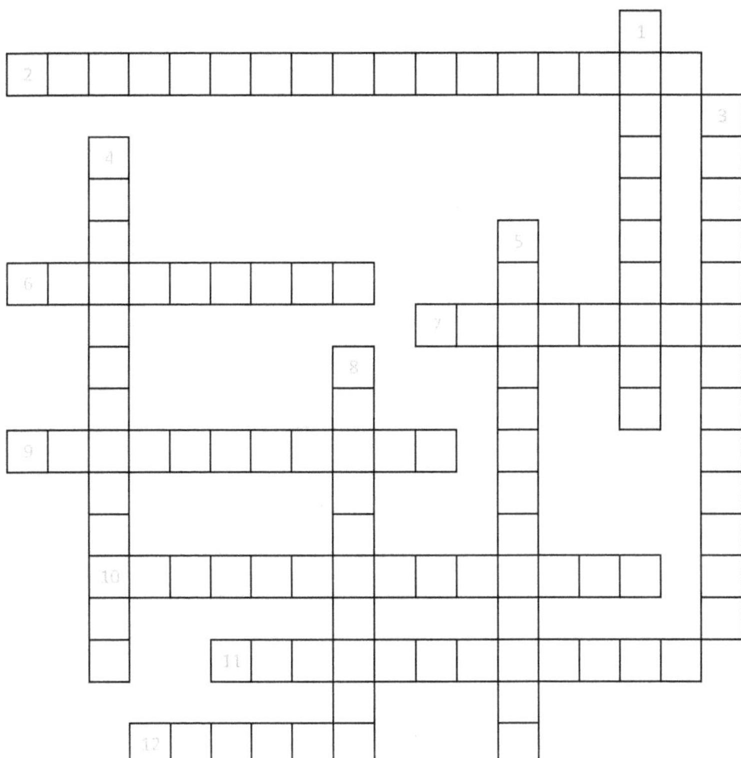

Across

2. Criteria's that makes a subject ineligible for participation in a clinical trial.
6. Time period and storage condition under which a drug is stable.
7. Refer to time scale.
9. A therapy that alters the genetic structure of cells for treating genetic diseases.
10. Letter issued by the EC or regulatory agencies granting the approval for conduct of a clinical trial.
11. An effort to devise in silico simulations of human physiology and genetic variation, to identify compounds that will eventually fail in the drug development process.
12. _________ requirements must be fulfilled for a valid EC meeting.

Down

1. Individual identifier based on physical characteristic such as a fingerprint, thumb impression, retina scan etc.
3. A technique for modeling and building libraries of chemical compounds for consideration as drug candidates ____________ Biosynthesis.
4. The care provided to patients when they are admitted to a hospital or health care center.
5. Refers to a system of making experimental drugs available to individuals, who are unable to participate in clinical trials.
8. The act of copying someone's words, ideas, results and presenting them as original content.

Crossword # 53

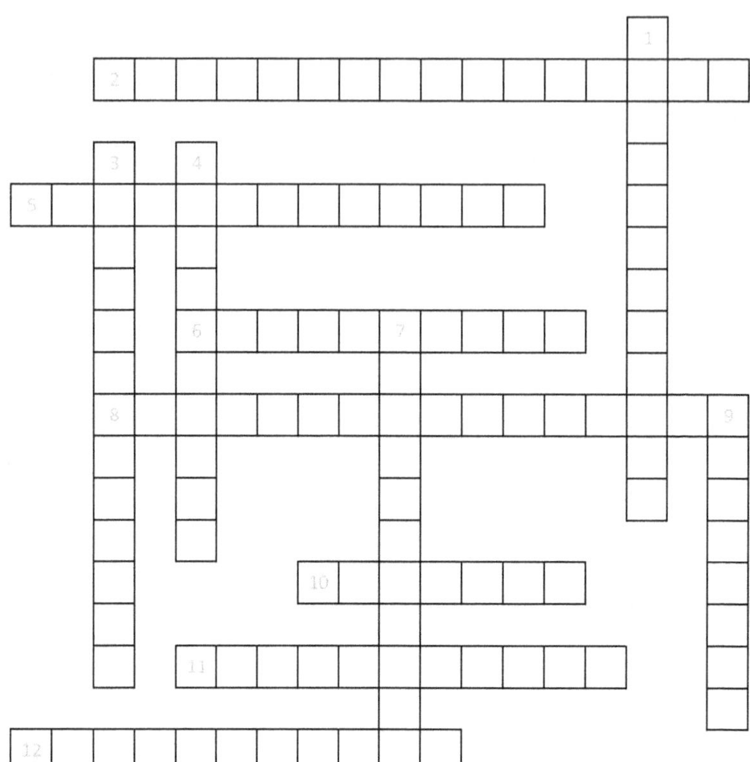

Across

2. A clinical trial design in which investigational product is compared with an approved drug or placebo.
5. Yearly summary reports submitted to EC or regulatory agencies on the progress of a trial.
6. Refers to the release of protected health information of a study subject, by one entity to another entity.
8. Review of planned matrices versus actual figures.
10. Trials conducted after drug's efficacy is demonstrated, but prior to regulatory submission of NDA.
11. Submission of documents to regulatory authorities via computer files.
12. The act of enrolling subjects according to the inclusion/exclusion criteria.

Down

1. Large stocks of clinical trial supplies.
3. Report prepared after interim analysis of data.
4. A document to demonstrate that a procedure, process and activity will consistently lead to the expected results ____________Certificate.
7. Clinical ___________ refers to the noting or record of clinical signs and symptoms in a subject.
9. The genetic constitution of an individual is known as _______________.

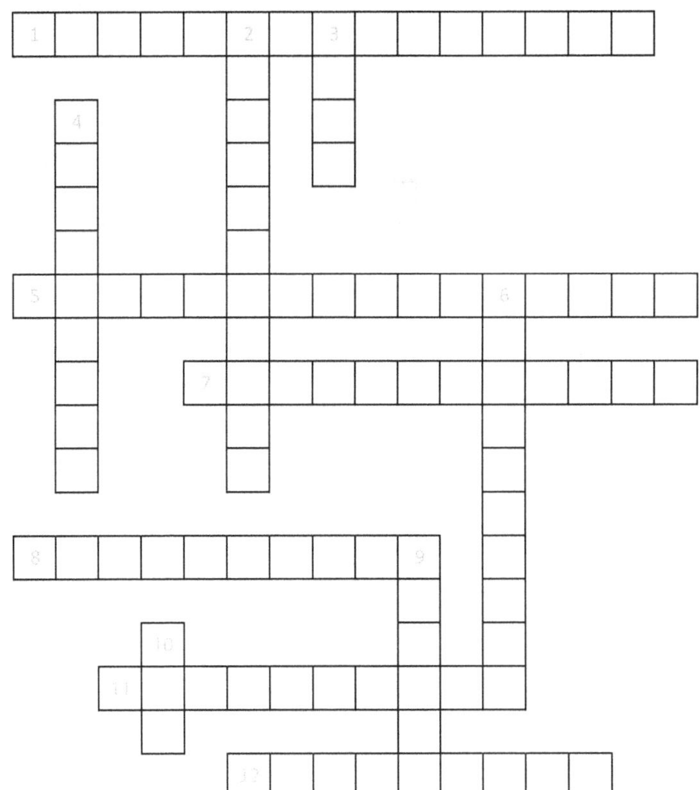

Across

1. At preclinical testing the regulatory bodies generally ask for_______________ profile of drug.
5. The entity responsible for the pharmacological action of a drug substance.
7. Normal value ranges for standardized laboratory tests.
8. Refers to the pharmaceutical delivery system for a drug product.
11. The process of collecting, recording and summarizing data that is collected from experiments, records and survey.
12. Individuals who participates in a phase-1 clinical trial or a BA/BE studies.

Down

2. A written evaluation of the audit results by the auditor.
3. A federal government agency that issues assurances and oversees compliance of regulatory guidelines by research institutions.
4. Minimal concentration level at which a drug is able to produce an effect in human body is called minimum ___________ dose.
6. Forms/documents containing study specific information, required to be filled in by the study subjects.
9. _______ survival time refers to the time at which 50% of the study population is alive.
10. Clinical trial exemption is commonly denoted as _________.

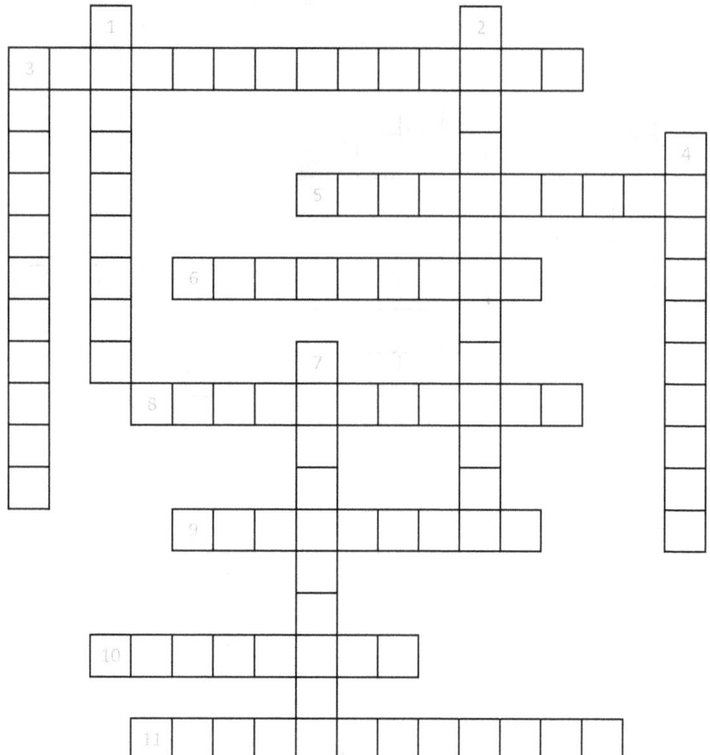

Across

3. A document that characterizes the data content of a system.
5. Ability to act on one's own behalf, after having understood all the consequences thereon.
6. Refer to discovery of a new drug, device,method, process or useful improvement upon any of these.
8. US-FDA regulations on electronic records and electronic signatures.
9. A person who provides social, emotional, medical and financial support to an individual.
10. Time required to eliminate 50% of the drug from the body.
11. Payment made to the study subjects for participation in a clinical trial.

Down

1. An investigational product or marketed product or placebo used in a clinical trial.
2. A result or finding which suggests the presence of an observation, which turns out not to be there.
3. A dosage form that contains one or more drug substances.
4. Large scale clinical trials having a sample size of 10,000 or more that evaluates the marginally effective investigational product.
7. A clinical trial that address new methods of preventing disease is known as ____________ trial.

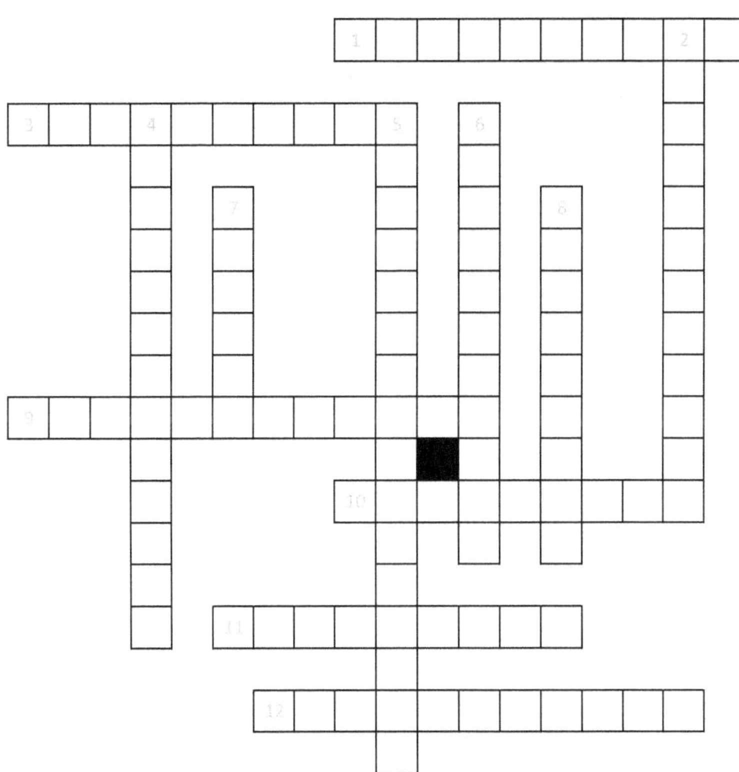

Across

1. ___________ Intervals represents a plausible range for the population value results from the sample.
3. An archival media on which essential trial documents can be transferred at a very small size.
9. Constitution of study team at a trial site is the responsibility of _______________.
10. __________Trial refers to a clinical trial designed to examine the benefits of a product in real-world environment.
11. Replacing a document with the new one after the same has been revised/ updated.
12. The process of matching one set of data elements, to their closest equivalents in another data set or in a reference dictionary.

Down

2. An extremely serious and expensive health problem that could be life threatening or may cause lifelong disability.
4. ___________study is based on historical data already existing in the records.
5. A clinical study designed to demonstrate the efficacy of a product.
6. A designation of the FDA to indicate a therapy developed to treat a rare disease.
7. A process by which a child provides his/her willingness to participate in a clinical trial.
8. A display of the shape of distribution for numeric variables useful for examining a

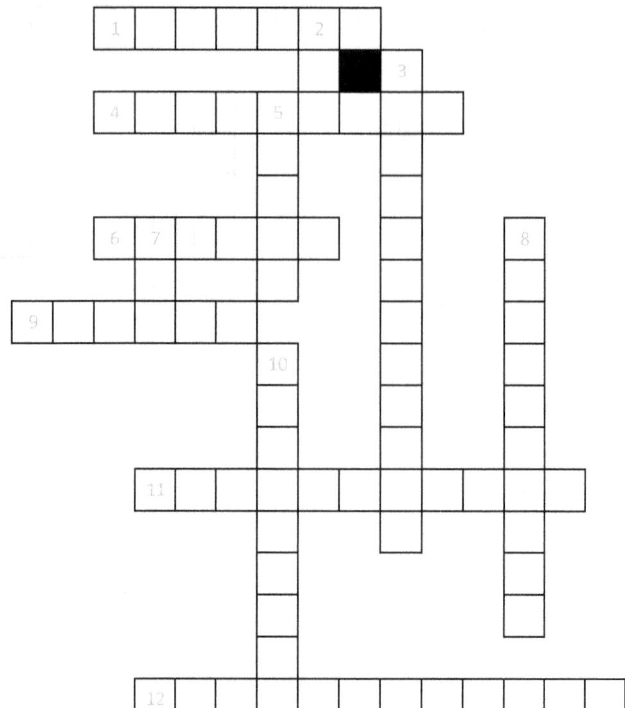

Across

1. A program designed to give supportive care to people in the final phase of a terminal illness either at home, independent facilities or within hospitals.
4. A strategy employed in clinical trials comparing two treatments, where each patient receives both the treatments, one followed by other.
6. Clinical investigation studies in subjects with the target disease, to determine efficacy, safety and tolerability in carefully controlled dose-ranging studies.
9. Therapeutic Exploratory Trials.
11. _______ _________Analysis is done to quantify the benefits associated with the use of a particular medication vis-à-vis direct cost implications.
12. The Science of drug and their clinical use is called clinical______________.

Down

2. An independent entity, contracted by the sponsor to conduct drug development services on its behalf.
3. Time frame for reporting SAEs to IRB/EC as per Schedule-Y_____ _______Days.
5. Time frame for reporting fatal or life-threatening unexpected ADRs to regulatory agencies as per ICH-GCP (no later than)_______Calendar Days.
7. A drug discovery approach that involves testing the potential drug substances against the target using automated robotic techniques.
8. A set of rules for streamlining processes according to a set routine.
10. The year in which Declaration of Helsinki came in force 19_________.

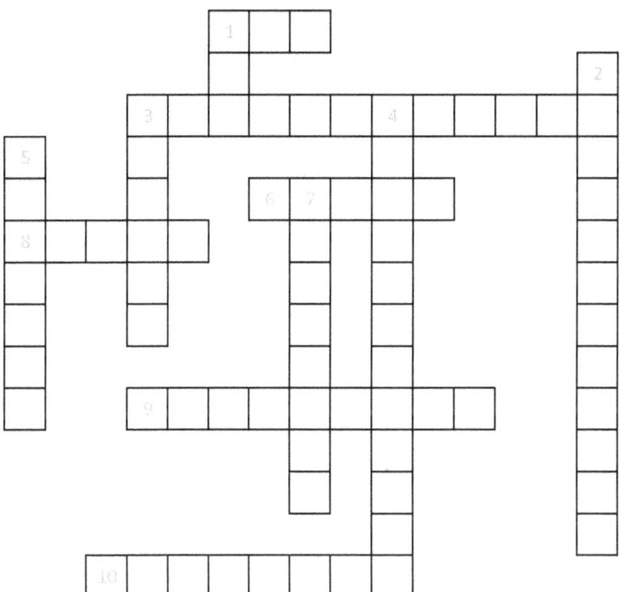

Across

1. An ICH defined format for regulatory submission that is considered acceptable in Japan, Europe, US and Canada.
3. The study of the effect of drugs on living organisms.
6. One of the aims of GLP is to help reduce the incidence of ________positive results.
8. An act causing physical, social or mental harm or discomfort.
9. Refer to the level of fluid in human body.
10. Time required to eliminate 50% of the drug from the body.

Down

1. A document signed and dated by investigator and the sponsor of a trial, describing the responsibility, timelines, payment schedule and other relevant terms.
2. A single legal entity that uses or discloses protected health information only for a part of its business operation.
3. Final pre-marketing phase of a clinical trial.
4. An estimate of the total cost implication for carrying out a particular activity.
5. Trials conducted after drug's efficacy is demonstrated, but prior to regulatory submission of NDA.
7. A brief summary including the objectives, methods, results and conclusion of a clinical trial or any other research work.

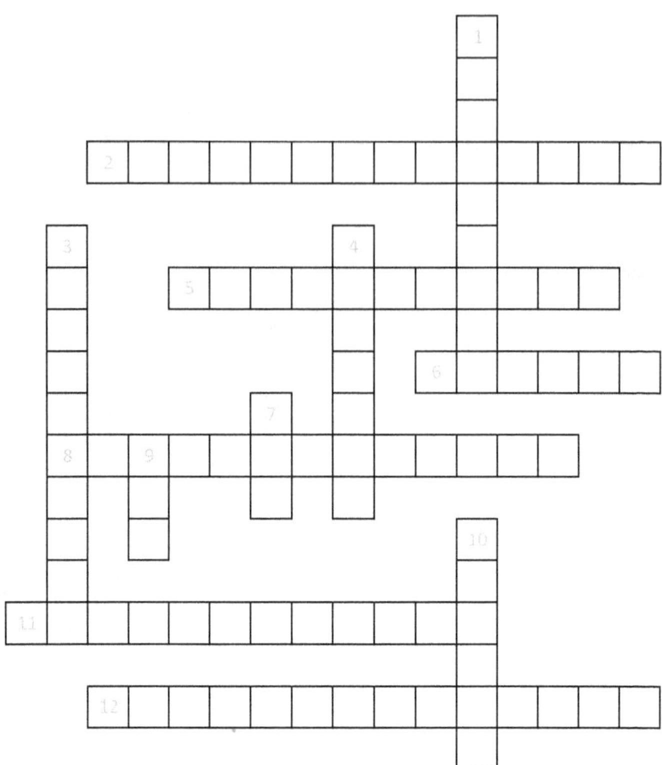

Across

2. Letter issued by the EC or regulatory agencies granting the approval for conduct of a clinical trial.
5. Refers to the testing of experimental drugs in the test tube or in animals before trials in humans can be carried out.
6. Tests conducted inside the body of a living organism.
8. A mechanism by which the access to clinical trial facility or documents is restricted to authorized individuals.
11. Primary object of a clinical trial (e.g. drug, vaccine, behavior, device or procedure).
12. The process of verifying the data entered in the case report form against the source data in order to establish its accuracy and completeness.

Down

1. Refer to intentionally misleading or withholding information.
3. Refers to a condition that forms the basis for the initiation of a treatment or of a diagnostic test.
4. A part that is a definite fraction of a whole sample for laboratory testing or analysis.
7. A written, dated and signed agreement between two or more parties that sets out arrangements on delegation and distribution of tasks, obligations and if applicable on financial matters.
9. A notification under __________ scheme is required for all clinical investigation use of a product in Australia.
10. An element of chance or having no specific pattern.

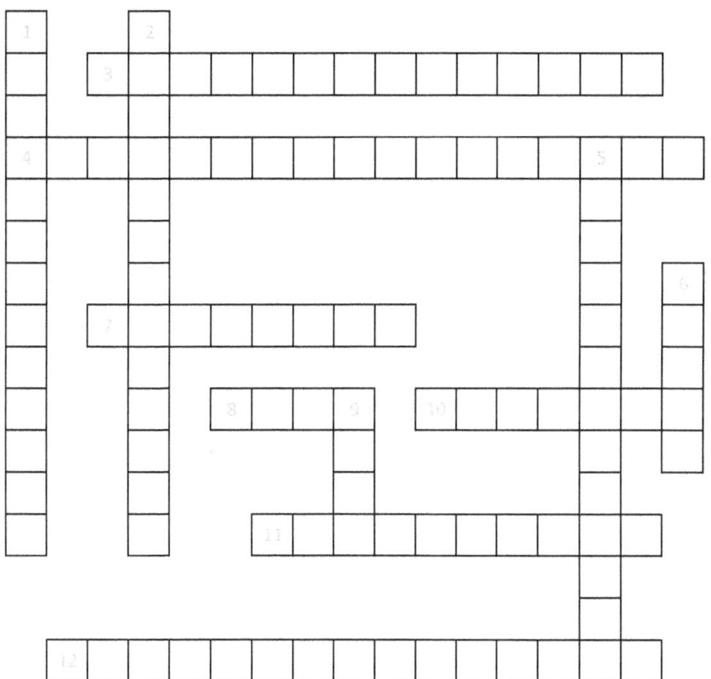

Across

3. Refer to organizational hierarchical structure of the supervisors and the subordinates.
4. A person who assists the Investigator in the conduct of research project.
7. An amendment in the existing documents or processes.
8. An independent data monitoring committee established by the sponsor to periodically assess the progress of a clinical trial, the safety data, and the critical efficacy endpoints.
10. A process of submitting competitive proposals to a trial sponsor.
11. A substantial disruption of a person's ability to conduct normal life functions.
12. Adverse event in which a subject is at immediate risk of dying.

Down

1. ___________study is based on historical data already existing in the records.
2. Investigation of an approved drug in a new/unapproved indication.
5. Permission to use and share a subject's protected health information for the purpose of a research study.
6. Articles (other than food), intended for use in the diagnosis, cure, mitigation, treatment or prevention of disease in man or other animals.
9. A preconceived personal preference or inclination that might influence the assessment of the trial.

Crossword # 61

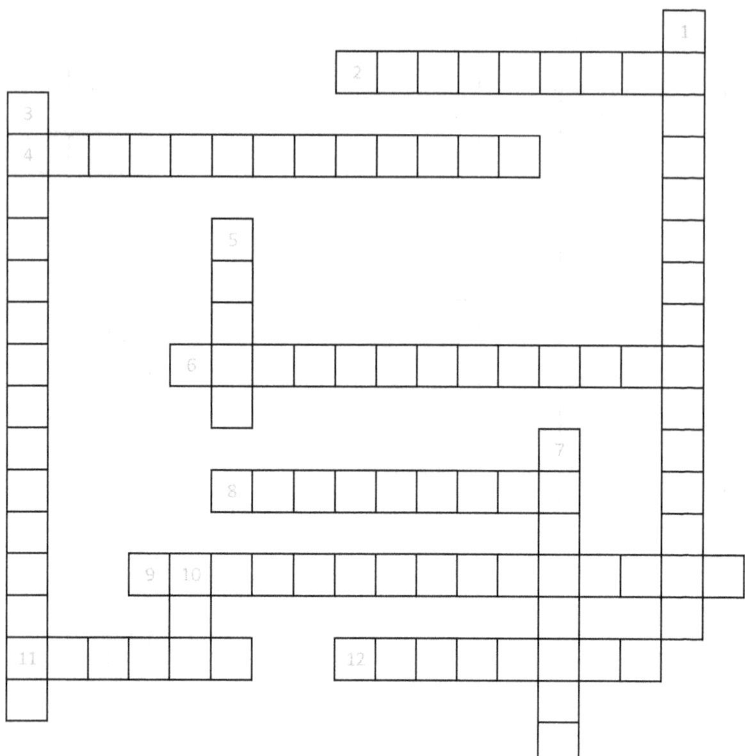

Across

2. Term used for a potential drug substance.
4. Description of the circumstances in which a particular data is required.
6. Number of new events in a population during a specified period of time.
8. Minimal concentration level at which a drug is able to produce an effect in human body is called minimum ____________ dose.
9. Target Selection is being revolutionized through the application of ______________.
11. Written instructions or rules to achieve uniformity, consistency and decision making.
12. The ability to understand the purpose, procedures, risks, benefits and alternatives to a research study.

Down

1. Technique involving genetic linkage studies and genetic association studies.
3. Therapy provided to the patient in order to prevent the disease recurrence after the primary therapy has shown complete response.
5. The physical abnormalities that are linked to an adverse event.
7. Intensity of an adverse event.
10. An environment in which trial data is directly entered into a web based data management system.

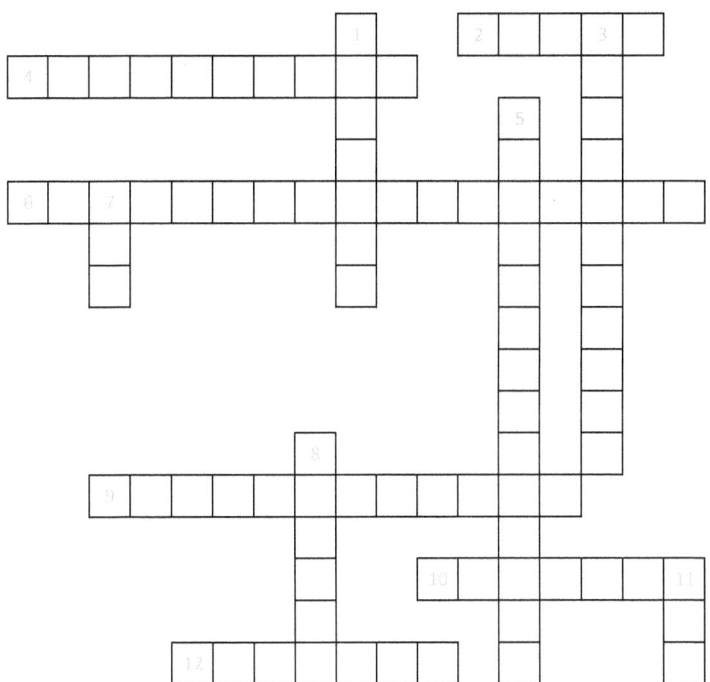

Across

2. ANDA does not require incorporation of animal and ________ data to establish safety and efficacy.
4. Complexation influences ____________ of a drug.
6. Criteria that makes a subject eligible for a clinical trial.
9. An effort to devise in silico simulations of human physiology and genetic variation, to identify compounds that will eventually fail in the drug development process.
10. Pilot clinical trials to evaluate safety in selected patient populations.
12. Controlled trials to evaluate safety and efficacy for determining a dose range to be studied in Phase-3 trials.

Down

1. Concentration/strength of a drug, at which it is effective.
3. Sign, symptom or laboratory results, not characteristic of normal individuals.
5. A document that characterizes the data content of a system.
7. Written description of the outcome of a trial.
8. Investigational New Drug Application is filed to initiate the testing of a drug in __________.
11. Noxious and unintended response to medicinal product at any dose.

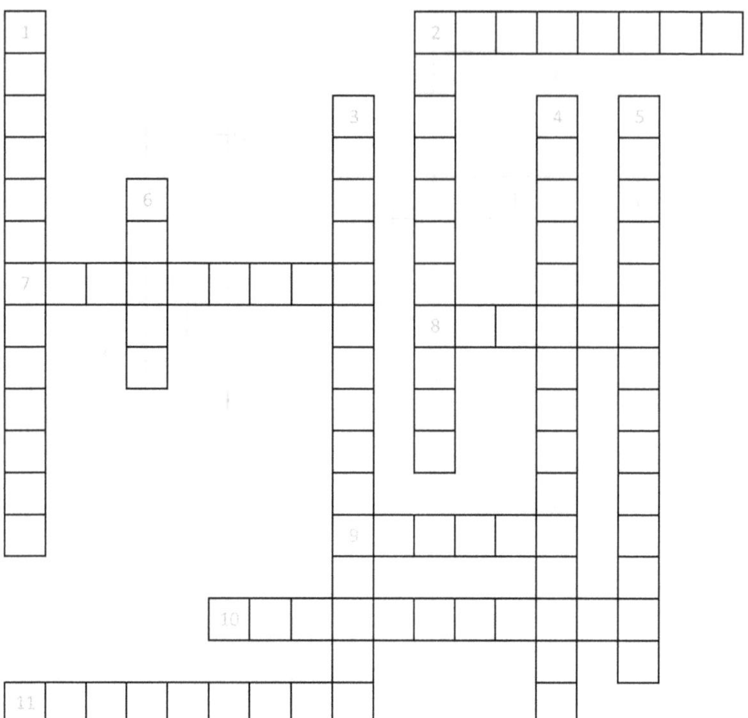

Across

2. Process of converting the data entered in an electronic data entry system to 'read only' format.
7. A step by step procedure for making a series of choice, among alternative decision to reach an outcome.
8. Sponsor-FDA meeting held to discuss the presentation of data (both paper and electronic) in support of the drug application.
9. A list of topics to be discussed in a meeting.
10. ____________ statement is signed by investigator(s) at the end of the trial to document their compliance with ICH-GCP and applicable regulatory requirements.
11. The closeness with which results replicate analyses of a sample.

Down

1. A scale for ranking items where the distance between adjacent points are equal.
2. The process of matching one set of data elements, to their closest equivalents in another data set or in a reference dictionary.
3. A legal statement or document indicating protection or exemption from liability for compensation of damages from a third party ____________letter.
4. A legal statement or document indicating protection or exemption from liability for compensation or damages from third party.
5. The process of handling the data collected during a clinical trial.
6. A person authorized to act on behalf of another person.

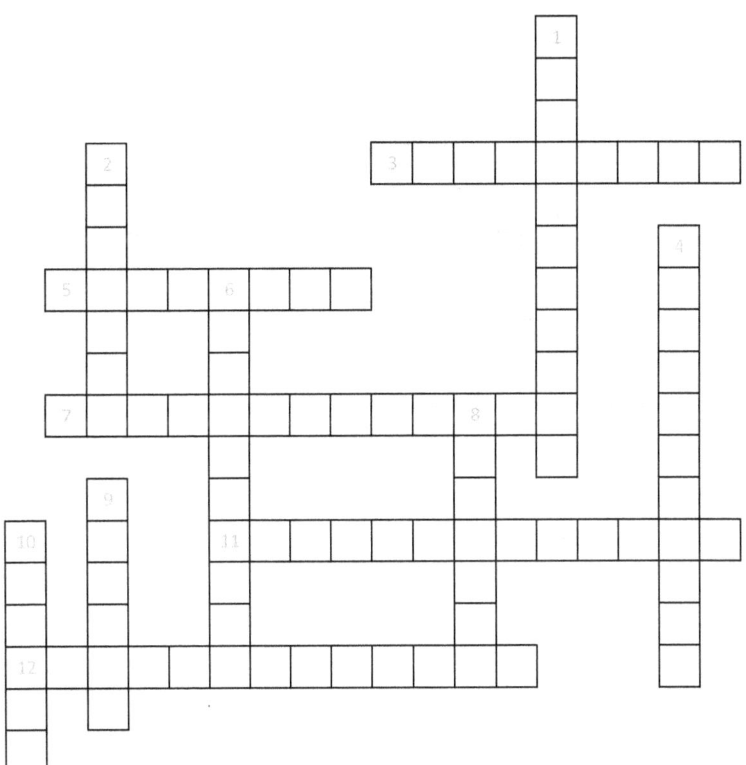

Across

3. Type-2 statistical error.
5. Systematic investigation designed to develop new/innovative products, processes or services as well as improvisation of the existing products, processes or services.
7. A list published on US FDA's website containing the names of personnel that have been disqualified from conducting clinical trials on grounds of medical fraud.
11. New Drug Application is filed to obtain marketing ____________.
12. A drug discovery approach that involves finding a drug or group of drugs which works on the selected targets.

Down

1. Discovery by chance.
2. Official or legal permission to an individual or organization by a competent authority to engage in a practice, occupation or activity.
4. Actual cost associated with an activity.
6. Action letter from the regulatory agency after review of a NDA, which signals that the drug can be approved. ________________ letter.
8. Non clinical testing conducted in an artificial environment (such as a test tube or culture medium).
9. __________ requirements must be fulfilled for a valid EC meeting.
10. A standardized dictionary of medical terminology adopted by the ICH.

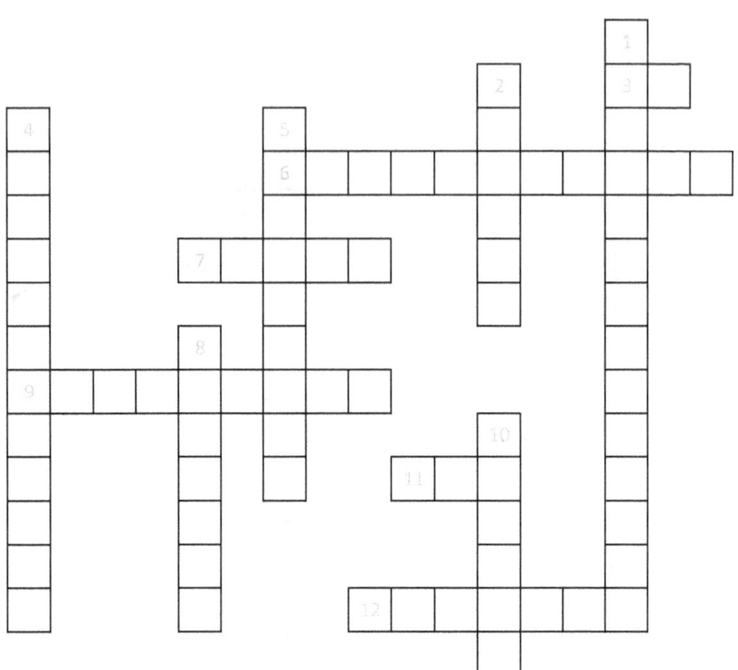

Across

3. Guidelines for Statistical Principles.
6. A quality control process of standardizing the equipment, machines, apparatus to be used in scientific testing.
7. Refers to an individual who has not attained the legal age of consenting to a trial, as per the applicable regulations.
9. Ethical principle of assigning patient to different arms, where the clinician does not have any preference for one arm over the others.
11. Any untoward medical occurrence that at any dose results in death or hospitalization or disability or congenital anomaly or is life-threatening.
12. The body of a deceased person used for imparting medical education.

Down

1. A medically qualified personnel in an organization who supports the marketing and/ or research department.
2. A computer that acts as a gateway for providing one or more services over a computer network.
4. Data to represent situations where the event of interest (e.g. survival, death, response etc.) is not recorded for a patient.
5. The study of cost-benefit ratio of drugs with other therapies or with similar drugs is known as Pharmaco________________.
8. The responsibility of filing NDA (New Drug Application) to the regulatory authorities lies with_________.
10. _______ Survival Time refers to the time at which 50% of the study population is alive.

Crossword # 66

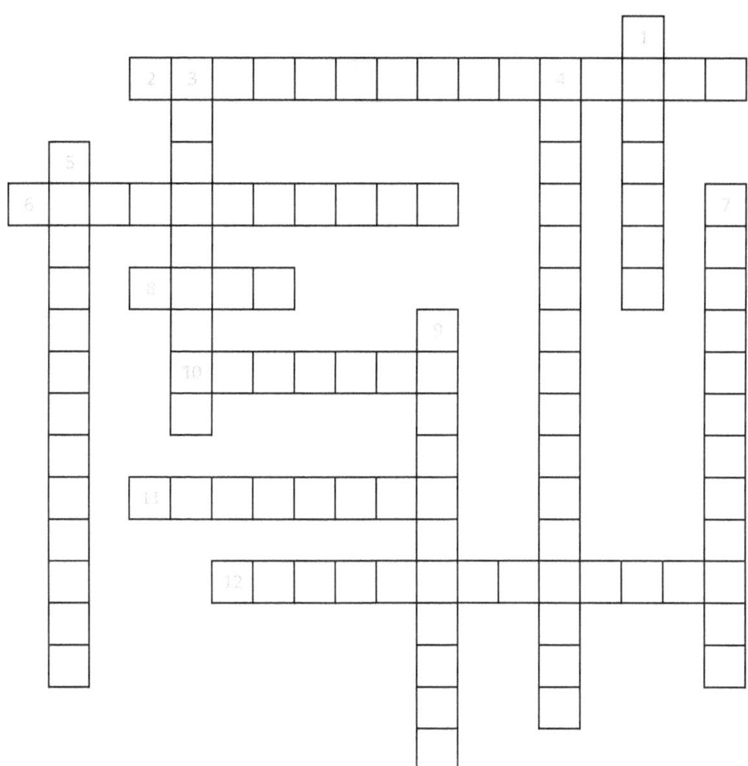

Across

2. Central value from a series of observation around which all other observations are dispersed.
6. Any public or private entity or medical or dental facility where clinical trials are conducted.
8. Most frequently occurring value in a set of data.
10. The responsibility of the preparation and submission of Regulatory Dossier lies with __________.
11. An electronic platform that contains the data generated from a clinical trial.
12. Statistical principle which states that all randomized patients should be included for analysis.

Down

1. Preclinical testing is mainly done on __________.
3. Refers to a stage of being balanced or in equilibrium.
4. Process of checking the accuracy of the data that has been entered into a computer database.
5. Yearly summary reports submitted to EC or regulatory agencies on the progress of a trial.
7. A preventive measure.
9. A written plan to define the critical project milestones, cost estimate, timelines and deliverables.

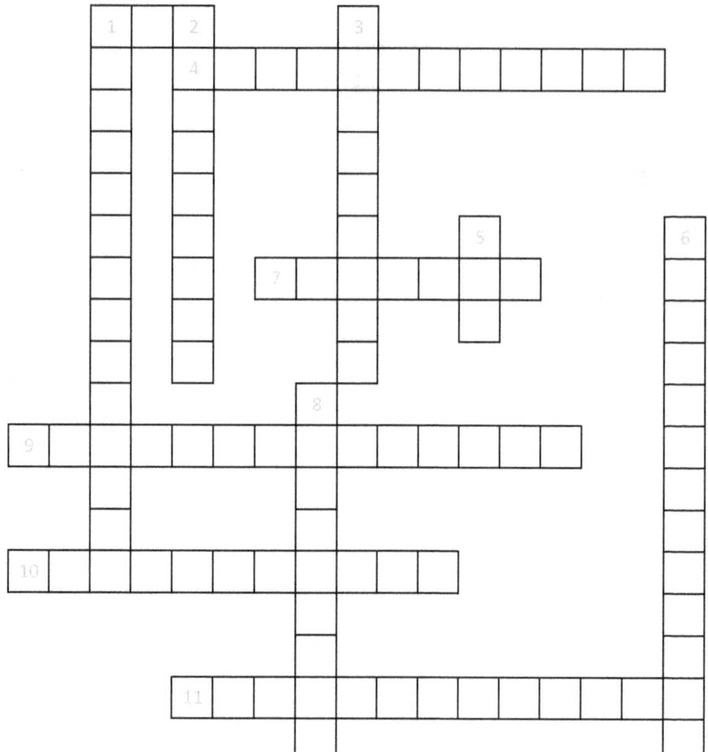

Across

1. Application filed to regulatory agencies for initiating phase I trial .
4. Any untoward medical occurrence in a patient, who has been administered an investigational product and which does not necessarily have a causal relationship with the treatment.
7. The concentration of a drug at which it is effective.
9. The category of drugs that undergo parallel track review by FDA.
10. The extent to which tests or procedures assess the same characteristic, skill or quality is known as Internal ___________
11. A document used for subject recruitment after obtaining EC approval that contains non-coercive trial information.

Down

1. Title 21 of the CFR, Section 312 covers _________.
2. Errors in either collection or recording of clinical trial data.
3. _________Trial refers to a clinical trial designed to examine the benefits of a product in real-world environment.
5. A document generated to resolve the data query on a particular page of CRF.
6. The accuracy and validity of a given data.
8. ___________ health information refers to any information about health status, provision of health care or payment for health care that can be linked to an individual.

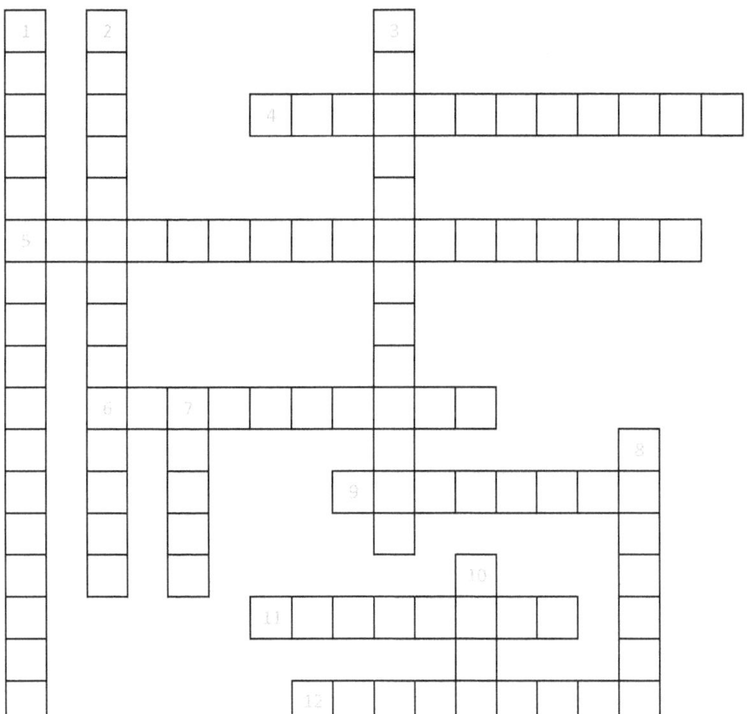

Across

4. An environment in which the access to trial related information is not controlled.
5. Toxicological testing (up to 9 months) in two species of animals to determine the effect of drug on fertility and reproduction.
6. The documentation of activities that allows reconstruction of the course of events.
9. A compilation of the clinical and non clinical data on the investigational product(s) is known as Investigator's____________.
11. A document that describes the objective(s), design, methodology, statistical considerations and organization of a trial.
12. A person who submits a trial application to a regulatory agency.

Down

1. A document that set forth the payment terms in a clinical trial.
2. The process whereby one determines the clinical meaning or significance of data, after the relevant statistical analysis have been performed.
3. A validated data collection form that contains a series of questions to assess an individual's response on a topic/parameter.
7. A fatal outcome of an adverse event.
8. Achievement of a desired outcome in a clinical trial.
10. Regulatory Authority responsible for regulating clinical trials in India.

Crossword # 69

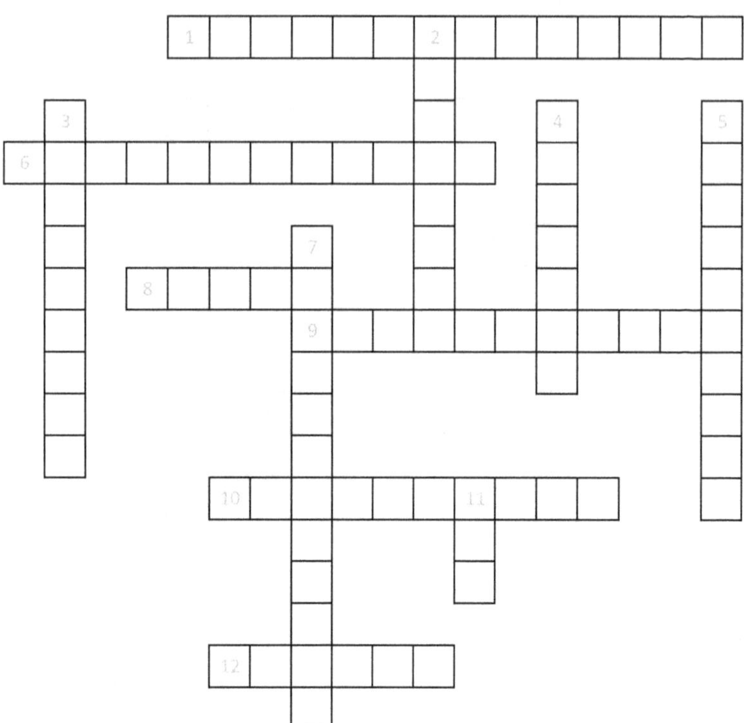

Across

1. Original documents, data and records.
6. A log that captures the dates of enrolment and other protocol required visits of a clinical trial subject.
8. Storage area on a computer's hard drive where the web page and/or graphic elements are stored temporarily.
9. A dosage form that contains one or more drug substances.
10. Characteristic of a drug used to determine crystal morphology and particle size.
12. Sequence of instructions that are interpreted or carried out by another program.

Down

2. Procedure for breaking the treatment codes in a blinded clinical trial.
3. The act of signing up participants into a clinical study.
4. Stakeholder responsible for the supervision, coordination and execution of successful data management of a clinical trial.
5. An objective or goal to be achieved in a stipulated time-frame.
7. Safety narratives prepared from serious adverse events.
11. Person who provides technical and statistical programming related expertise and advice.

Crossword # 70

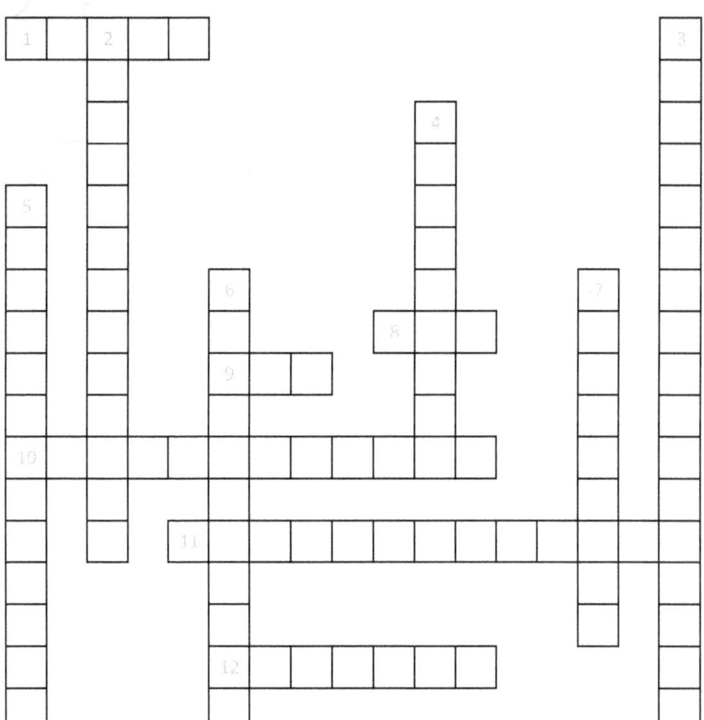

Across

1. Regulatory body headed by DCGI.
8. Document that establishes agreement between two or more parties for ensuring the confidentiality of information provided by one party to the other.
9. Application filed to regulatory agencies for obtaining marketing authorization of a new drug.
10. The branch of medical science that deals with the study of incidence, distribution and control of a disease in a population.
11. Written description of the outcome of a trial enumerating the clinical and statistical interpretations:-________ ______Report
12. The responsibility for the creation of essential trial documents like Protocol, ICF, and IB etc lies with________.

Down

2. Primary or secondary outcome(s) used to judge the effectiveness of a treatment.
3. Investigator is responsible for obtaining the ERB/IEC approval of the trial at a __________.
4. An investigational product or marketed product or placebo used in a clinical trial.
5. Refers to an event or outcome to answer the primary hypothesis of a clinical trial.
6. The extent of harm or discomfort anticipated from a clinical trial which is not greater than the routine practice.
7. Refers to the waivers that are provided under special circumstances with appropriate documentation of authorization.

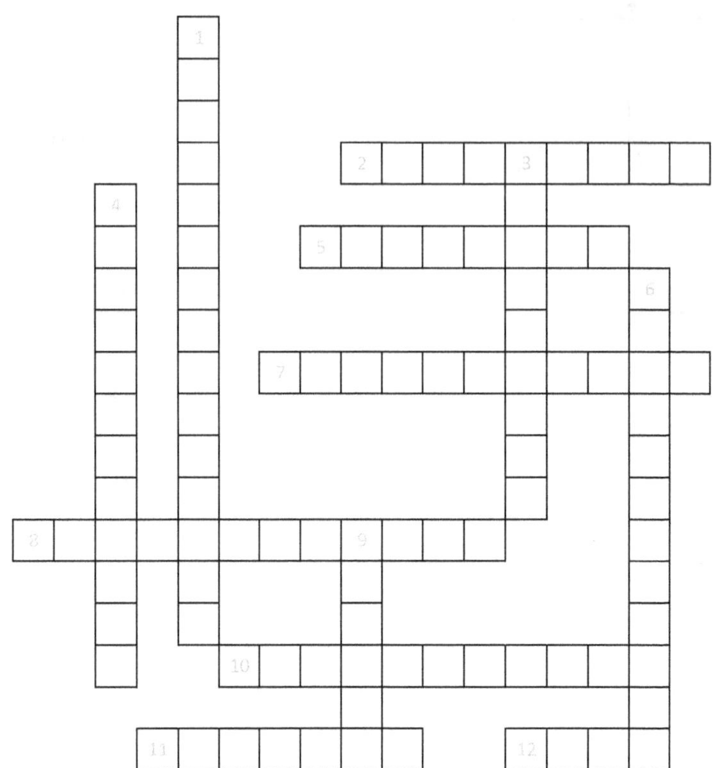

Across

2. Non compliance to either protocol schedule of events or standard operating procedures.
5. A written description of a work plan.
7. A variable that is based on categorical data and cannot be measured numerically.
8. Constitution of study team at a trial site is the responsibility of ________________.
10. Accelerated approval is also known as Accelerated ____________.
11. A pre-set standard for measuring the outcome.
12. A comparison of case report form and ancillary data to the raw data in the clinical trial reporting database for the purpose of demonstrating the accuracy of data process.

Down

1. Statistical analysis of trial data at a predefined time interval before all subjects has completed the trial.
3. A formal written, binding commitment.
4. Yearly review of the progress of a trial by ethics committee(s) or regulatory agencies.
6. All the SAEs should be personally signed by ____________.
9. A process by which a child voluntarily confirms his/her willingness to participate in a clinical trial.

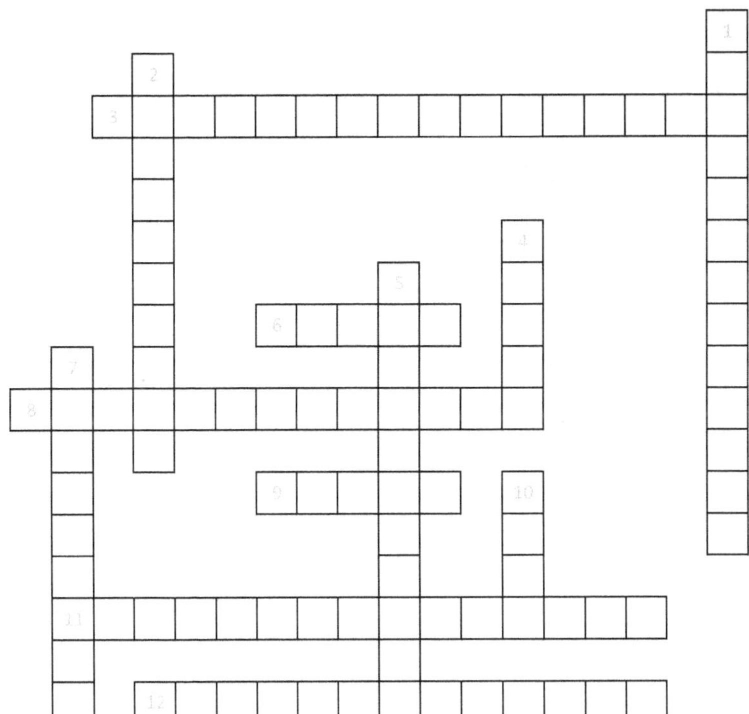

Across

3. An electronic signature based upon cryptographic methods of originator authentication such that the identity of the signer and the integrity of the data can be verified.
6. Forms/documents containing study specific information, required to be filled in by the study subjects.
8. Report prepared after interim analysis of data.
9. A systematic and Independent examination of trial related activities and documents.
11. A type of non-commercial IND.
12. A comparison of case report form and ancillary data to the raw data in the clinical trial reporting database for the purpose of demonstrating the accuracy of data processing.

Down

1. A validated data collection form that contains a series of questions to assess an individual's response on a topic/parameter.
2. Cognitive impairment refers to a medical condition in which an individual's capacity for judgment and reasoning is significantly____________.
4. A systematic and independent examination to determine whether trial related activities were conducted and the data were recoded, analyzed and accurately reported according to protocol.
5. Ownership of sole rights of a document, process or product.
7. De-identified information of a trial participant that in no way can disclose his/her identity.
10. A comparison of CRF and ancillary data to the raw data in the clinical trial reporting database.

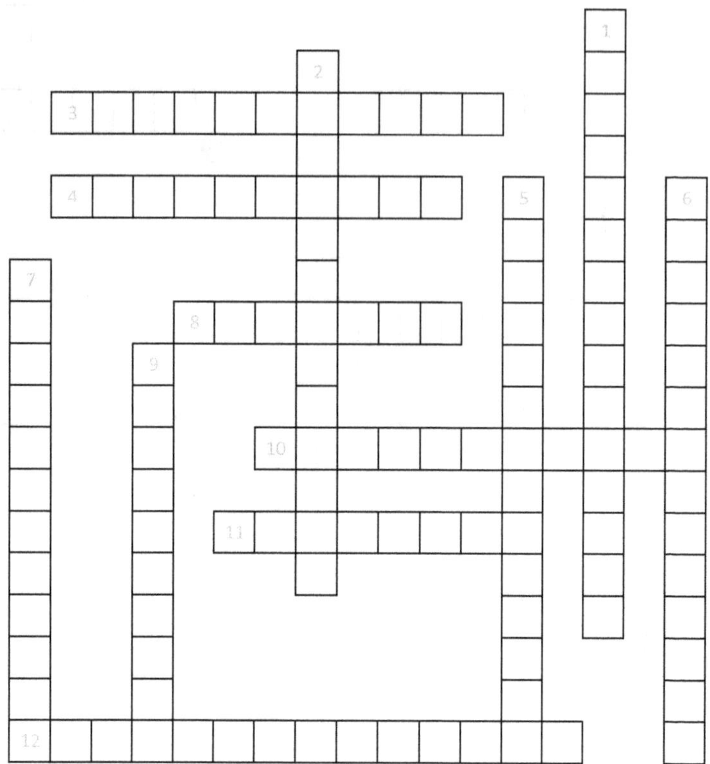

Across

3. A process of estimating the magnitude of some attributes of an object such as its length or weight.
4. All information in original record and certified copies of original records of clinical findings, observations or other activities in a clinical trial.
8. Three basic ethical principles: respect for persons, beneficence and justice. ___________Report.
10. A written evaluation of the audit results by the auditor.
11. An event or outcome to answer the primary hypothesis of a clinical trial.
12. A patient, who does not meet the inclusion criteria, falls under the category of _________.

Down

1. A type of non-commercial Investigational New Drug Application submitted by a physician who both initiates and conducts an investigation and under whose immediate direction the investigational drug is administered or dispensed.
2. Compounds identified via High Throughput Screening process.
5. An Individual or juridical or other body authorized under applicable law to consent on behalf of a prospective subject for participation in a clinical trial.
6. Refer to pharmacokinetics of a drug substance.
7. Large stocks of clinical trial supplies.
9. An archival media on which essential trial documents can be transferred at a very small size.

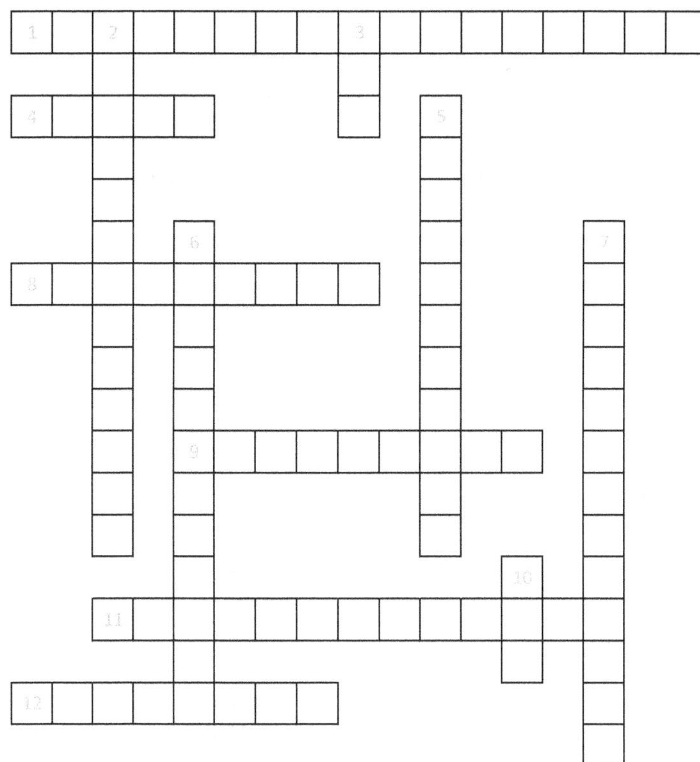

Across

1. Criteria's that makes a subject ineligible for participation in a clinical trial.
4. An organization responsible to develop and support global platform-independent data standards that enable information system interoperability to improve medical research and related areas of healthcare.
8. A subject who has satisfied the entire protocol requirements and is eligible for the safety and efficacy analysis.
9. Formal submission of a trial application by a sponsor to the regulatory agency, followed by obtaining no objection for initiating the trial is referred as Clinical Trial ____________.
11. Refers to the time period between the initiation and completion of a trial at a site.
12. The Treatment group of a clinical trial.

Down

2. Any investigation in human subjects intended to discover or verify the clinical, PK/PD, and adverse reactions of an investigational product.
3. The paper used in Case Report Form (CRF) for manual entry.
5. Methodology used to investigate a drug or device for its safety and efficacy.
6. Toxicity studies for 18-24 months in vivo and in vitro are done to assess ____________.
7. Closing a clinical study after the same has been completed or prematurely terminated/suspended.
10. A classification of regulatory inspection outcome that does not require any action or response.

Crossword # 75

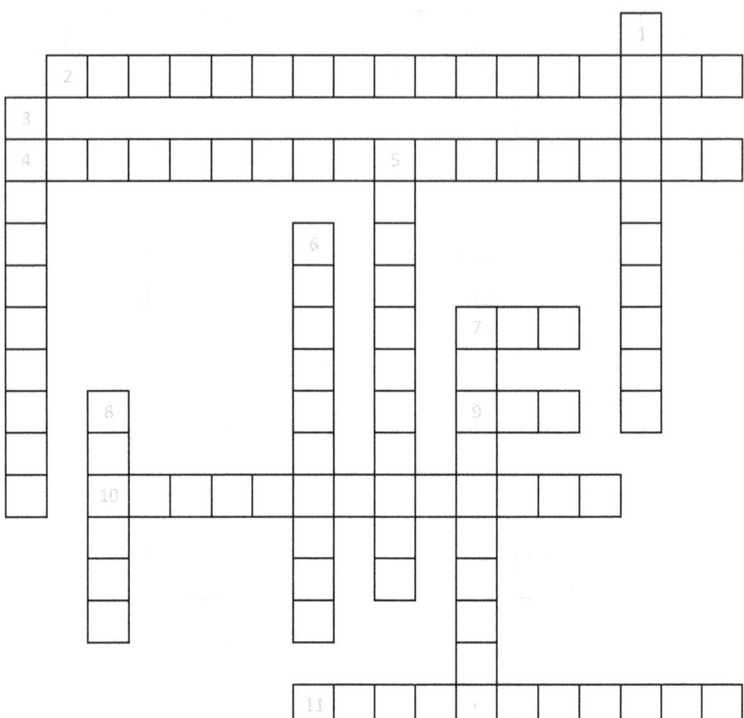

Across

2. A statistical test that provides an analysis of variance by ranks and is the non-parametric equivalent of the F-test for analysis of variance.
4. A non interventional study conducted according to routine medical practice.
7. Drug Regulatory Agency in USA.
9. Regulatory Agency in Australia.
10. Application filed primarily by companies, whose ultimate goal is to obtain marketing approval for the new product.
11. Substances or agents that can interfere with normal embryonic development.

Down

1. A government order with the force of the law.
3. Name of a website/web server.
5. Clinical ____________ refers to the noting or record of clinical signs and symptoms in a subject.
6. United States agreement to cover all Federal sponsored research by a common set of regulations.
7. An event resulting in death of a subject.
8. Process of making a copy of important data, onto a different storage medium.

Crossword # 76

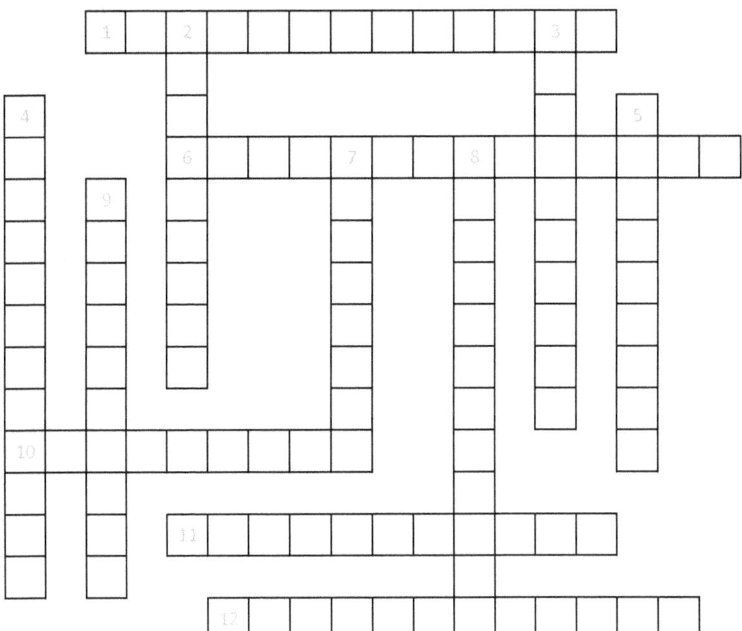

Across

1. A study in which a particular type of subject is equally represented in each study group.
6. A treatment designed to facilitate the process of recovery from injury, illness or disease to as normal a condition as possible.
10. Planned and systematic actions that are established to ensure that the trial is performed and the data are generated, documented and reported in compliance with GCP and applicable regulatory requirements is known as Quality_____________.
11. Investigator's assessment on the relatedness of an adverse event to the investigational product.
12. Payment made to the study subjects for participation in a clinical trial.

Down

2. A document that contains results of the laboratory tests.
3. Refers to the pharmaceutical delivery system for a drug product.
4. The allocation of specific trial related duties to the individual study team members at the investigator site is the responsibility of_____________.
5. Determination of the nature of a disease.
7. Measurements taken usually at the beginning of a study to serve as a reference for subsequent measurements.
8. Reporting of ongoing safety, progress reports, and re-approvals to IRB is the responsibility of___________.
9. Trials that are conducted to find better tests or procedures for diagnosing a particular disease or condition___________Trials.

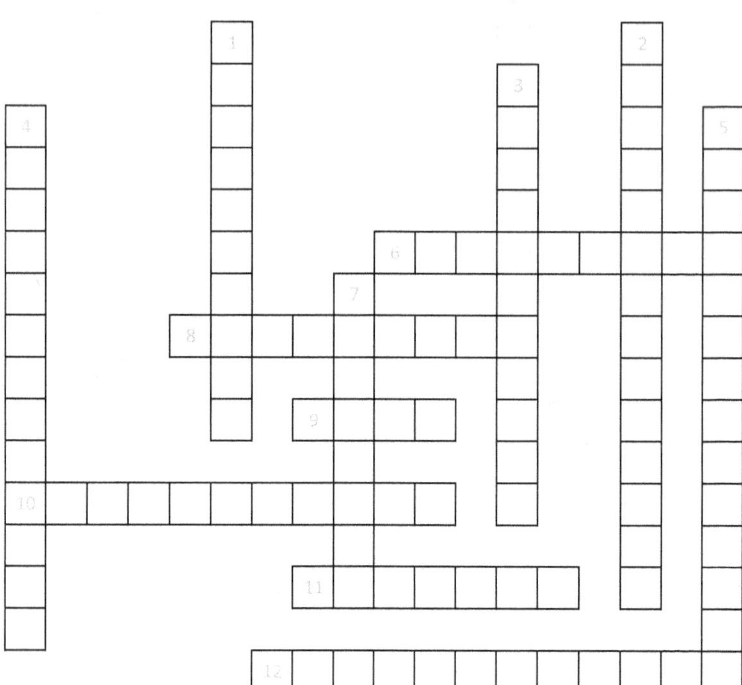

Across

6. A statistical approach in which patients are analyzed according to the treatment that they received, rather than the one to which they were randomized.
8. The period of time during which a woman is providing her breast milk to an infant or child.
9. An arithmetic value that is obtained by summing up all the observations and dividing by the total number of observations.
10. The design of a study in which neither the investigator nor the subject knows which medication the subject is receiving.
11. Respect for person, beneficence, justice are the three principles discussed in the ____________ Report.
12. Display of relation between two numeric variables while distinguishing between levels of categorical variables.

Down

1. Entry in the electronic case report form using a computer and modem through a distant location__________ ______Entry.
2. Operational techniques and activities undertaken within the quality assurance system to verify that the requirements for quality of the trial-related activities have been fulfilled.
3. A clinical trial in which two or more doses of an agent are tested against each other to determine which dose works best and is least harmful_______ __________ Study.
4. Refer to an article that has a potential to become a successful drug through systematic clinical trial investigations.
5. Hit compounds with suitable physical, chemical and biological properties.
7. Refer to pre-treatment evaluations on study subjects as they enter a clinical trial ____________Assessment.

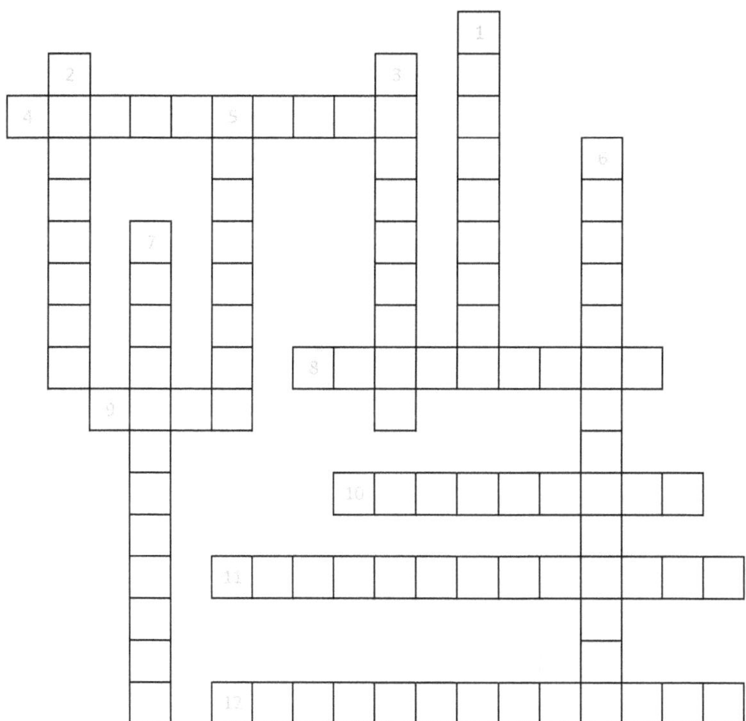

Across

4. All information in original record and certified copies of original records of clinical findings, observations or other activities in a clinical trial.
8. A type of in vitro and in vivo toxicological testing for 18-24 months to determine the mutagenic potential of a drug is known as ________Studies.
9. Animal species on which mutagenicity studies on a new product are conducted.
10. Drug Technical Advisory Board is the highest ___________ body, under Drug and Cosmetic Act 1940.
11. Recording of false data or results and reporting them.
12. Organization of European countries dedicated to increasing economic integration and strengthening cooperation among its members.

Down

1. Necessity of informed consent was first described in ____________ Code.
2. A type of statistical chart that displays information about the distribution of numeric variable.
3. The method by which the extent of relationship between a study drug and an adverse event is established is known as __________Assessment.
5. A process to ascertain that management of clinical trial(s) and associated processes, utilize qualified individuals is referred to as __________ Qualification Review.
6. A tool used during the randomization process to ensure an exact balance between the treatment arms with respect to key patient factors that are strongly related to the outcome variable.
7. The decision of regulatory authorities to put a clinical study on hold.

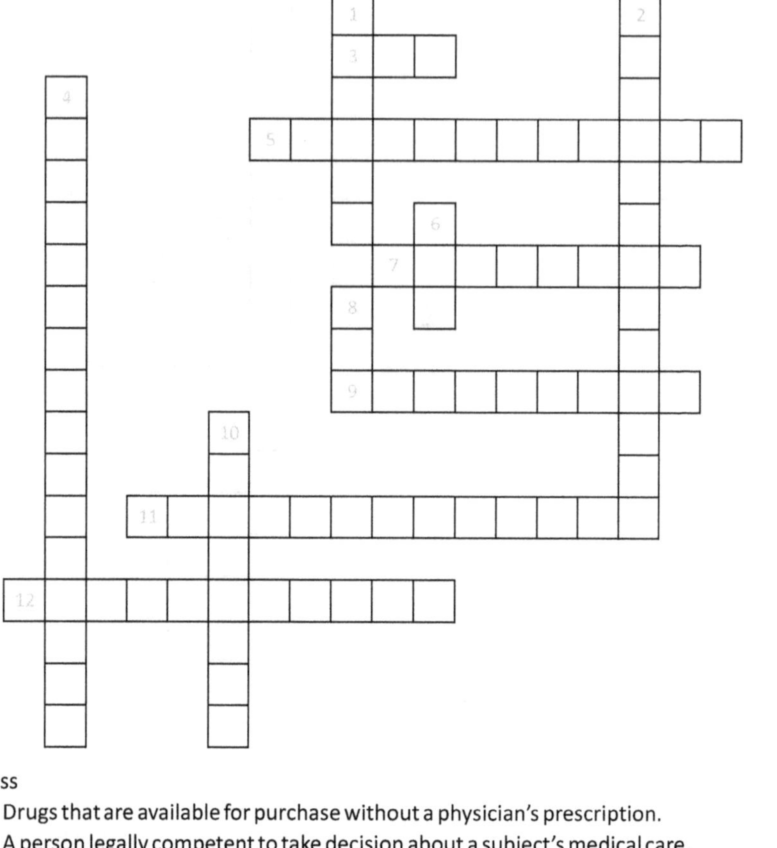

Across

3. Drugs that are available for purchase without a physician's prescription.
5. A person legally competent to take decision about a subject's medical care.
7. Relationship of significance in the life of a research subject such as parent-child, spousal, employer-employee ____________Relations.
9. The code of medical ethics, designed to protect the safety and integrity of study participants and which came as a result of medical experimentation conducted by Nazis during World War II__________________Code.
11. A technique for modeling and building libraries of chemical compounds for consideration as drug candidates_______________Biosynthesis.
12. The act of transforming document, text or phrases from one language to another.

Down

1. Permission to import the drug may be obtained by applying in _______ for a test license.
2. A technique of modifying an existing compound chemically to act on a selected target_______________Chemistry.
4. Medication taken by a study subject for diseases/medical conditions other than the study disease.
6. A classification of regulatory inspection outcome where official action is indicated.
8. Number of principles in Nuremberg Code.
10. A pre-designed form/document that includes standard fill-in-the-blank spaces for capturing the standard information.

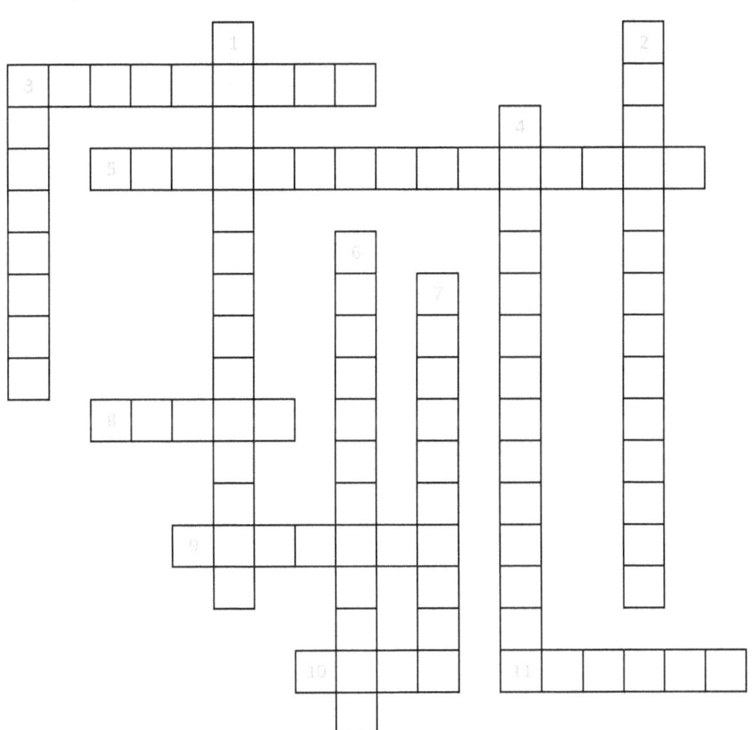

Across

3. Refer to the mock runs for any activity or process, before performing it in a real time environment.
5. Studies conducted to estimate the rate and extent of drug absorption.
8. Aerosols are used to deliver the drug in __________.
9. The result of an activity, process, investigation or intervention.
10. The main purpose of Phase-1 studies is to establish a _______ dosage range.
11. Down coding or down grading is part of _____________ audit.

Down

1. The arm in a clinical trial refers to ____________.
2. A patient who is no longer in touch with the site person/site during the trial.
3. Refer to time scale.
4. Information systems for analysis of genomic data.
6. Application for permission to conduct clinical trials for New Drug/IND in India is made in __________.
7. ____________ Intervals represents a plausible range for the population value results from the sample.

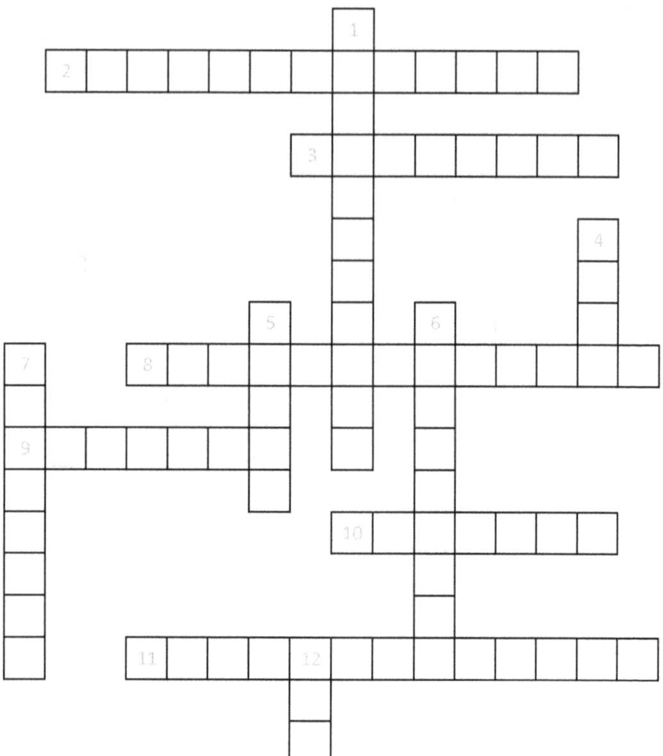

Across

2. Report prepared from a serious and unexpected adverse experience.
3. A type of statistical chart that displays the distribution of levels of a categorical variable.
8. Refers to the amount of a drug product to be administered at each specific dosing time.
9. A pattern of black vertical lines containing the coded information to uniquely identify and/or track clinical supplies.
10. Blinding is also known as ________.
11. Technique that uses living organisms, or substances from organism, biological systems, or processes to make or modify a product or process, to change plants or animals, or to develop micro-organisms for specific uses.

Down

1. The extent of relation between occurrence of an adverse event and administration of a drug/placebo.
4. The amount of a drug to be used for a medical condition.
5. A document for identifying a drug/placebo in compliance with applicable regulations and appropriateness of the instructions provided to the subjects.
6. The regression of a disease condition.
7. Federal Food and Drug Act in 1906 brought truth in ___________.
12. Guidelines for the choice of control group and related issue in clinical trials.

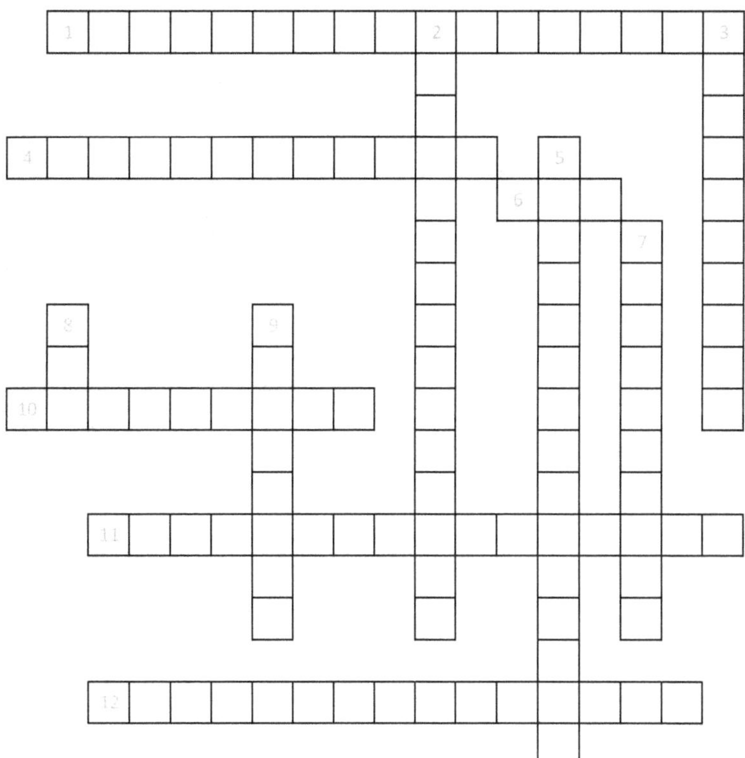

Across

1. Clinical trials conducted according to a single protocol at more than one site and by more than one investigator.
4. Combining the results of several studies that address a set of related research hypothesis.
6. Detailed, written instructions to achieve uniformity in the performance of a specific task/activity.
10. The relation of an adverse event (effect) to the study drug/procedure.
11. Review of planned matrices versus actual figures.
12. Compassionate use IND is also known as______________.

Down

2. Maintaining the minutes of EC meetings is the responsibility of___________.
3. An analysis involving a random variable.
5. Total surface area of the human body which is widely used for the calculation of drug dosages of cancer medicines.
7. Number of patients required to achieve the desired statistical significance in a clinical trial.
8. ICH Guideline on clinical safety data management.
9. Clinical study design in which one or more parties to the trial are kept unaware of the treatment assignment(s).

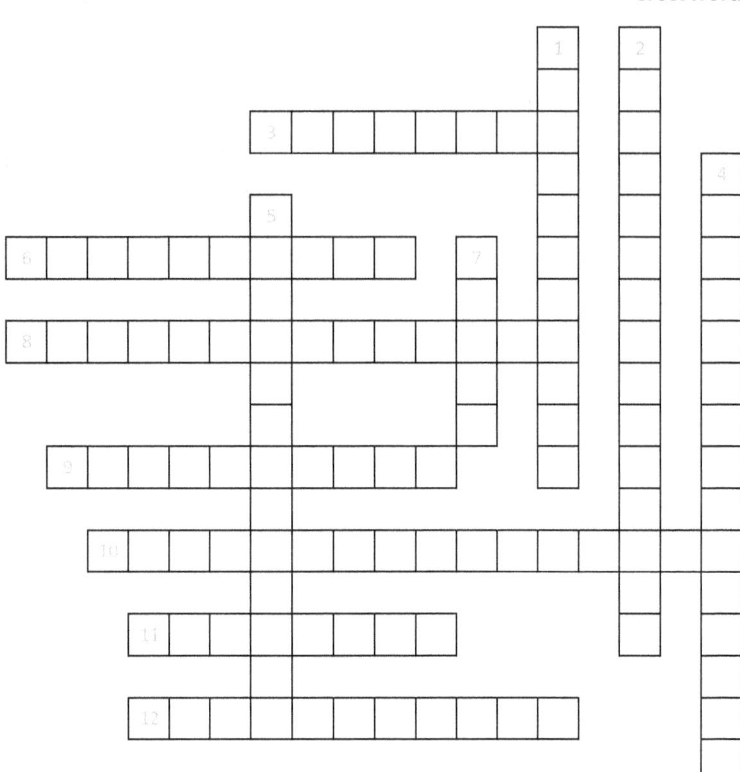

Across

3. Subsequent contact with a subject in order to assess current status of a subject's condition or outcome of an adverse event.
6. Adherence to study protocol, GCP guidelines and the applicable regulatory requirements.
8. An individual, who shares study responsibilities with the investigator at a trial site.
9. An organizational chart that describes different functional positions in an organization.
10. A measure of how a subject, feels, functions or survives.
11. An adverse effect produced by a drug that is detrimental to the participant's health.
12. Quantitative data such as number of patients, number of visits etc.

Down

1. A designation of the FDA to indicate a therapy developed to treat a rare disease.
2. A drug development approach that involves choosing a disease or biological target (such as enzyme, receptor, ion channel etc) to treat and then developing a model for that disease.
4. Studies that determines the maximum tolerated dose.
5. A result or finding which suggests the presence of an observation, which turns out not to be there.
7. Later stages of a developing organism (from conception to delivery).

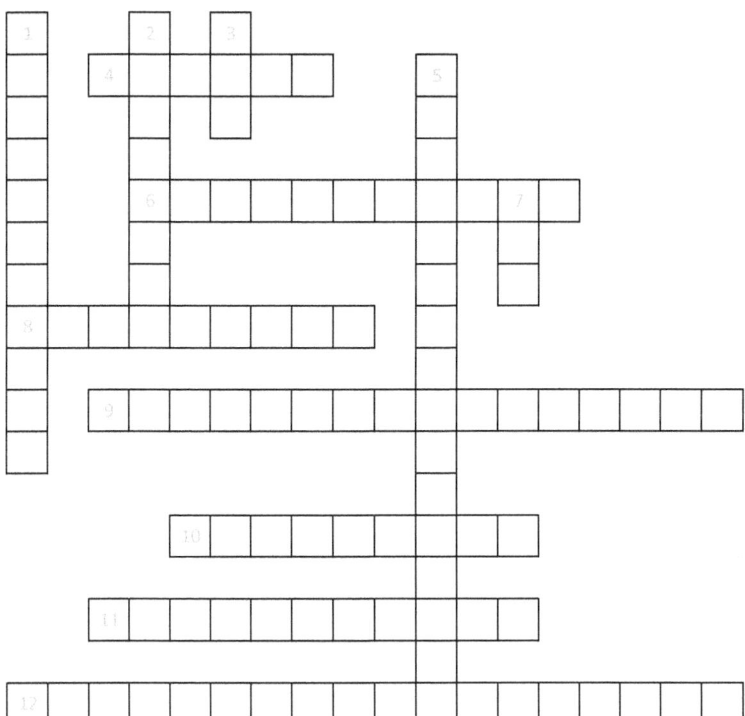

Across

4. Permission to carry out clinical trials with a new drug in India is issued in________.
6. A designation of the US-FDA to indicate a therapy developed to treat a rare disease.
8. A name, word, symbol or phrase used to identify a particular product.
9. Study of genetic variation underlying differential response to drugs.
10. Individuals who participates in a phase-1 clinical trial or a BA/BE studies.
11. A measurement of the strength of the relationship between two variables.
12. Individuals whose willingness to volunteer in a clinical trial may be unduly influenced in case of his refusal to participate.

Down

1. A measure of the strength of the relationship between two variables.
2. A chemical synthesized or prepared from natural sources that is evaluated for its biological activities in preclinical tests.
3. Practices required to be followed for the manufactured, handling and storage of Investigational Product.
5. Study of genetic variation leading to differential response to drugs.
7. A standard governing the manufacture of human and animal drugs and biologics intended to assure the quality and integrity of manufacturing data submitted to regulatory authorities.

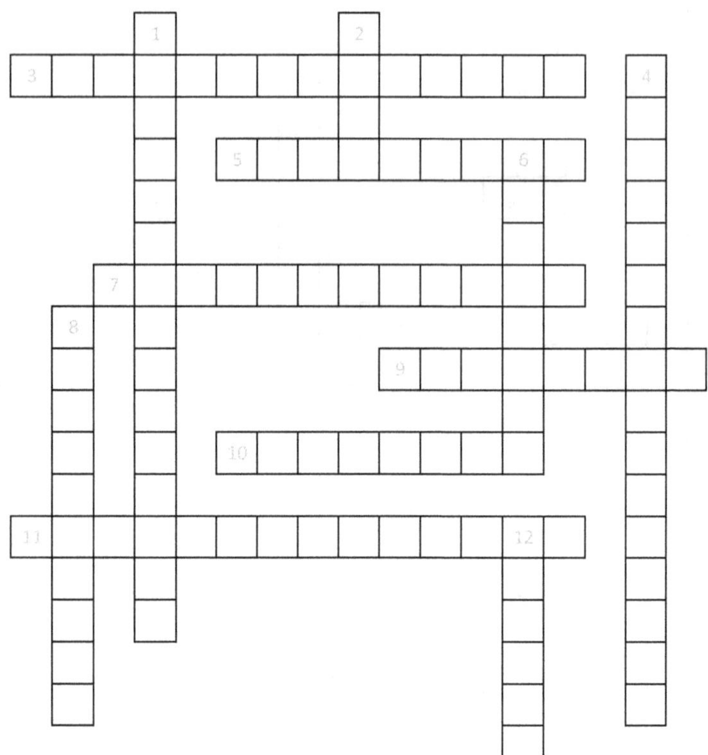

Across

3. The information on overall general health, past illnesses and current medical problems of a subject.
5. A person who provides social, emotional, medical and financial support to an individual.
7. Potential of a substance to cause cancer.
9. Pharmaco__________ refers to the physiological effect of drug on human body.
10. A product's ability to produce beneficial effects for a disease.
11. An authorization to undertake medical practice as per applicable regulations.

Down

1. The initial visit to investigator site by the sponsor/CRO personnel for evaluating the suitability of investigator and facility.
2. Facility for conducting clinical trials.
4. A biological molecule used as a marker to measure the progress of a disease or effects of a treatment.
6. A product's ability to produce beneficial effect on the course or duration of a disease.
8. Statistical Analysis is a part of clinical data __________ process.
12. Phase II of clinical trials evaluates the efficacy and ________.

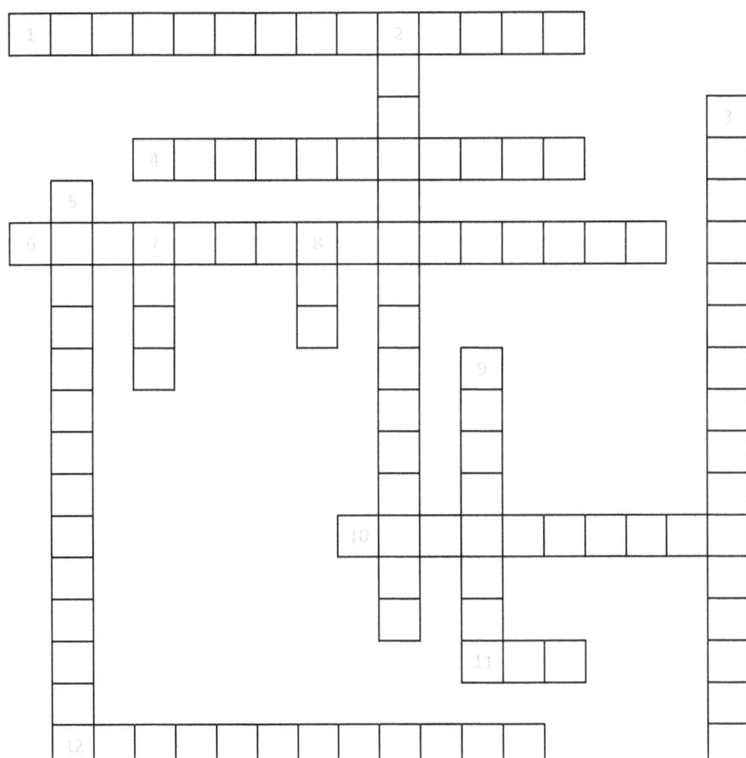

Across

1. A process of providing the health care services to an individual.
4. Articles published in peer-reviewed scientific journals.
6. Assessment of adverse events and serious adverse events experienced by the participants in a clinical trial.
10. Individual identifier based on physical characteristic such as a fingerprint, thumb impression, retina scan etc.
11. The Periodic Safety Update Report should be submitted every _______ months for first two years, after approval of drug is granted to the applicant.
12. Analysis that combines the results of several studies to address a set of related research hypotheses.

Down

2. A type of non-commercial IND.
3. A state in which a person is not able to manage his/her affairs or to make a choice due to a psychiatric or developmental disorder.
5. A printed, optical, or electronic document designed to record all of the protocol-required information on each trial subject.
7. Regulatory Agency for regulating clinical trials in Europe.
8. Organization responsible for managing the investigator sites in a clinical trial.
9. Study of the physiological effects of drug on human body is called Pharmaco _______________.

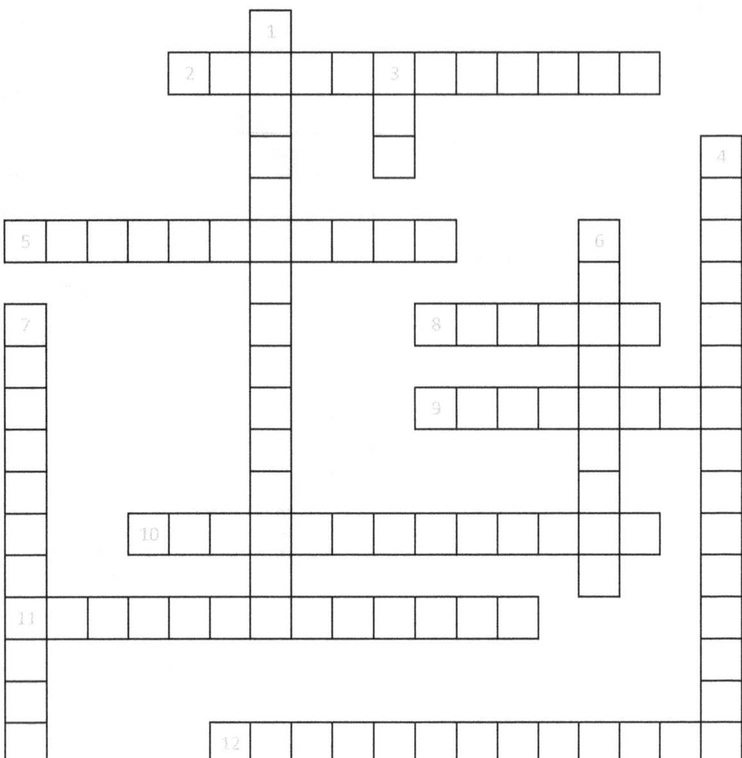

Across

2. An extremely serious and expensive health problem that could be life threatening or may cause lifelong disability.
5. Longitudinal studies in which the sample is a cohort.
8. Convenient and commonest drug dosage form.
9. Testing in human beings is known as _________ testing.
10. The total number of deaths relative to the total population at a specific place in a specific period of time.
11. A result or finding which suggest that an observation is not present but on further investigation is found to be present.
12. A subject matter expert in a peer-group.

Down

1. An independent body constituted of medical professionals and non medical members whose responsibility is to ensure the protection of the rights, safety and well being of human subjects.
3. A central file in which all the essential clinical trial documents are filed.
4. Official daily publication for rules, proposed rules and notices of federal agencies and organization in United States.
6. The absence of viable, contaminating microorganisms.
7. The notes to explain the deviation/ violation of a particular activity/ process.

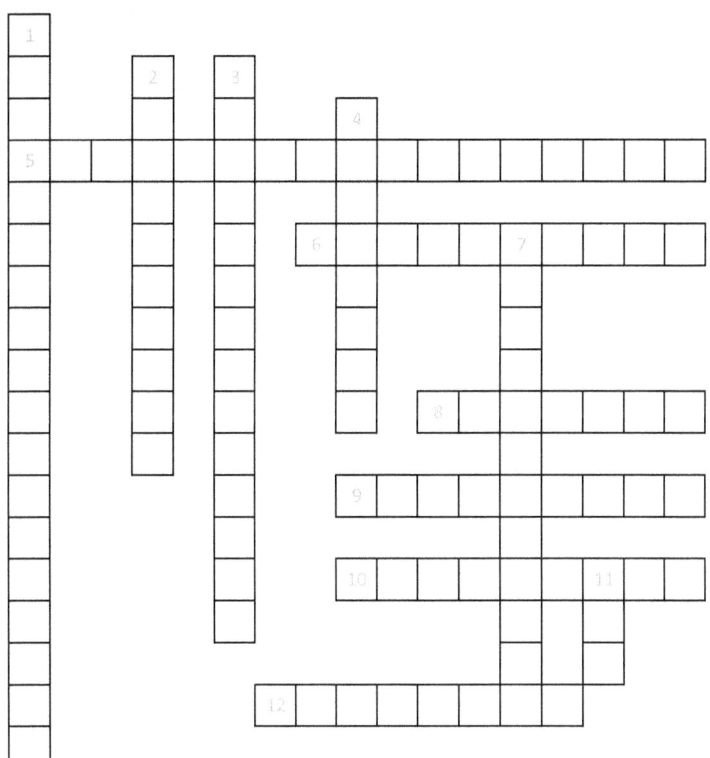

Across

5. Study of cost-benefit ratio of drugs with other therapies or with similar drugs.
6. The native language of a country or a place___________Language.
8. The number assigned to an essential document in use.
9. Pharmaco _______________ refers to methods of assessment and prevention of adverse events.
10. A law which excludes the users from using original works of authorship, fixed in any tangible medium of expression.
12. The genetic constitution of an individual is known as _______________.

Down

1. Authority that grants trial permission and monitors compliance with applicable regulatory guidelines.
2. Form 44 represents ____________ to conduct clinical trial in India.
3. The drug products that have the same active ingredient, dosage, form, route of administration, strength or concentration are as called ___________equivalents.
4. The study of genetic variation leading to differential response to drugs is called Pharmaco__________.
7. A comparison group of study subjects in a trial, who are not treated with the investigational agent.
11. A standard for the conduct and reporting of non-clinical laboratory studies intended to assure the quality and integrity of safety data submitted to regulatory authorities.

Crossword # 89

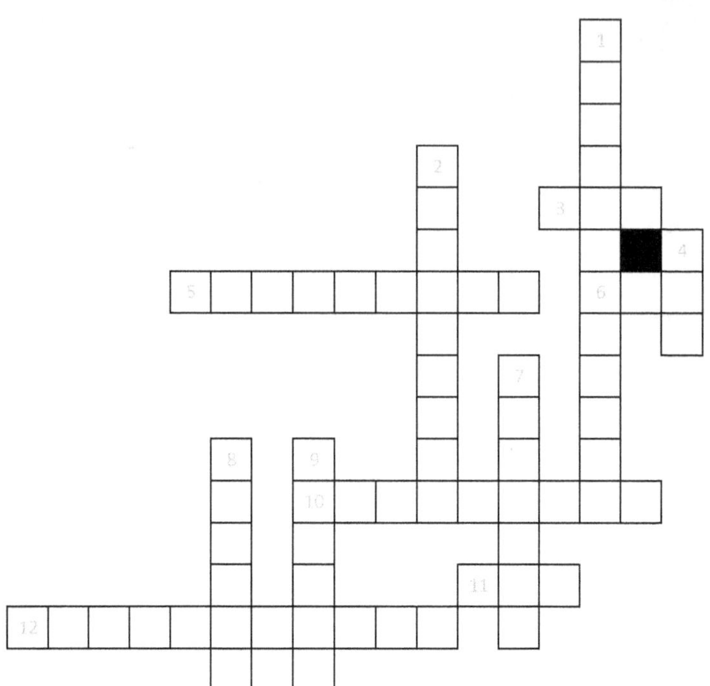

Across

3. Code of Federal Regulation is commonly denoted as ________.
5. Time period and storage condition under which a drug is stable.
6. Ancillary trial data is generally not collected on ___________.
10. A condition of being confined to home and requiring considerable efforts and assistance to leave the home.
11. A person or an organization contracted by the sponsor to perform one or more of a sponsor's trial related duties and functions.
12. Refers to the degree to which the results of studies included in a systematic review are similar.

Down

1. The act of making changes or amendments to an information, document or process.
2. Refers to a state of being fair, so that the benefits and burdens of research are fairly distributed.
4. An annual codification of the general and permanent rules published in the Federal Register (US), by the executive departments and agencies of the Federal Government.
7. Timeframe for reporting SAEs to sponsor.
8. Trial phase that evaluates the initial safety of a drug product.
9. Phase of the trial that involves healthy human volunteers.

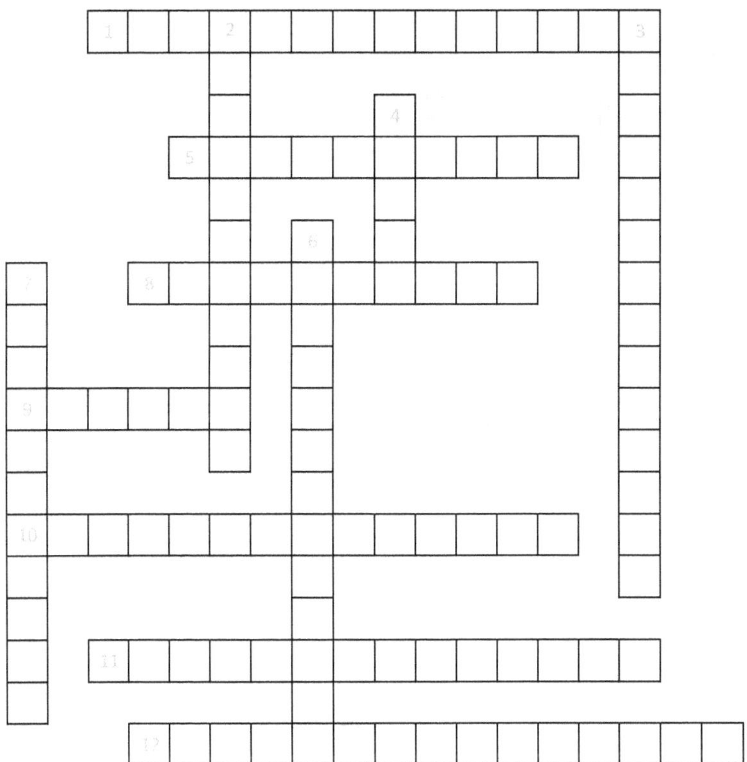

Across

1. Refers to pre-designed forms for recording trial data directly in to an electronic system.
5. Large scale clinical trials having a sample size of 10,000 or more that evaluates the marginally effective investigational product.
8. Review of facility and resources are the critical elements of clinical trial ______________.
9. Early stages of a developing organism (from conception to 8th week of pregnancy).
10. The process of assessing the readiness of an investigator site for initiating the enrolment in a clinical trial.
11. A file that contains all the essential trial documents at a trial site.
12. Biological timing and rythmicity that in human beings is characterized by cycles of approximately 24 hours.

Down

2. A type of retrospective study comparing persons with a given condition and persons without the condition with respect to antecedent factors______ ________________ Study.
3. A medically qualified personnel employed by trial Sponsor/CROs for reviewing critical medical data (safety and efficacy) of a clinical trial.
4. Any departure of the result from the "true" value is termed as ______________.
6. Data on the stability of a drug product under routine and accelerated stability conditions.
7. Complete records of patient's disease history entered in hospital files, out-patient charts or medical records.

Crossword # 91

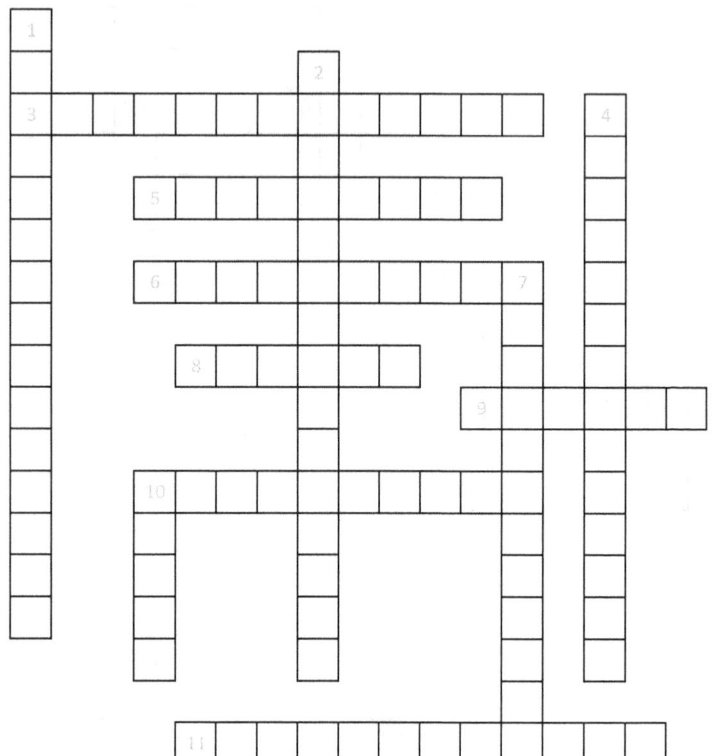

Across

3. A clinical trial database in which all the validation queries have been resolved and which is ready for analysis.
5. The frequency of disease, illness, injury, and disability in a population.
6. Codes used by the FDA to classify medical devices according to the potential risks or hazards.
8. A group of individuals identified on the basis of a common experience or characteristics that are usually monitored over time.
9. Conforming to an accepted standard of human behavior.
10. The process of collecting, recording and summarizing data that is collected from experiments, records and survey.
11. Normal value ranges for standardized laboratory tests.

Down

1. Trial design in which a special type of multi-arm trial allows more than one comparison to be carried out, without increasing the required sample size.
2. Advertisement for recruitment of study subjects require approval from ________.
4. A plan laid to define the monitoring visit intervals, source data verification requirements, protocol specifying monitoring instructions (if any) and other elements.
7. A person having knowledge and competence of statistics.
10. Suspected Unexpected Serious Adverse Reactions.

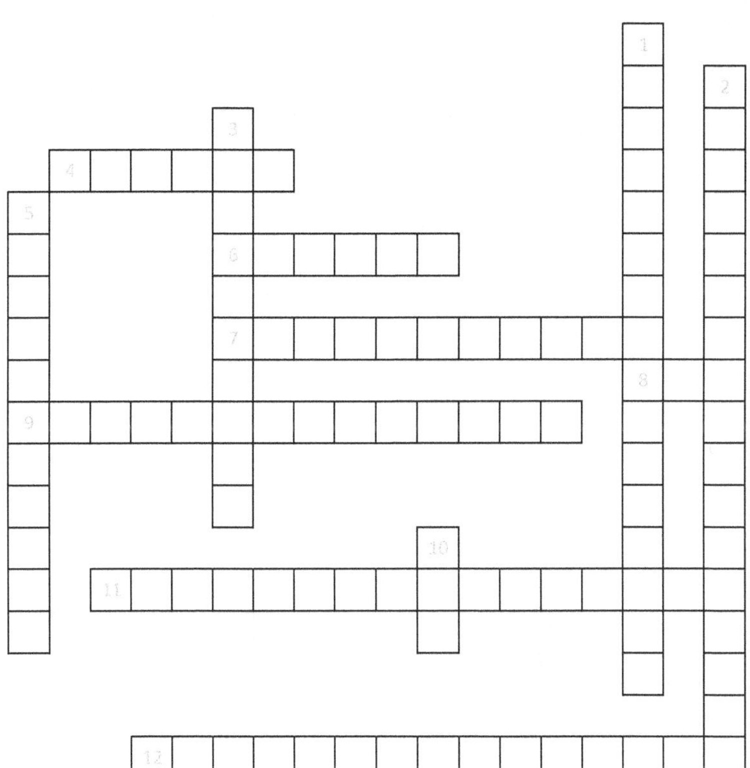

Across

4. A supplier of goods or services.
6. Human micro dosing studies, designed to speed up the development of promising molecular entities or imaging agents.
7. Timelines for the submission of a summary report in case of premature termination/suspension of a clinical trial.
8. An individual who shares study responsibilities with the investigator at the site.
9. Documents given to subjects for recording certain observations on the condition of their health, at their home or at trial site.
11. A specific circumstance when the use of certain treatments could be harmful.
12. A reference document that contains operating instructions for an equipment, activity or process.

Down

1. A screening test to identify if a person has an inherited predisposition to a certain phenotype, or is at risk of producing offspring with inherited diseases or disorders.
2. Use of available published data as a control arm.
3. Ability to act on one's own behalf, after having understood all the consequences thereon.
5. US-FDA regulations on financial disclosure by clinical investigators.
10. A form signed by the investigator and sub-investigators, to disclose their financial interest in the sponsor company, for whom they intent to participate in a clinical trial.

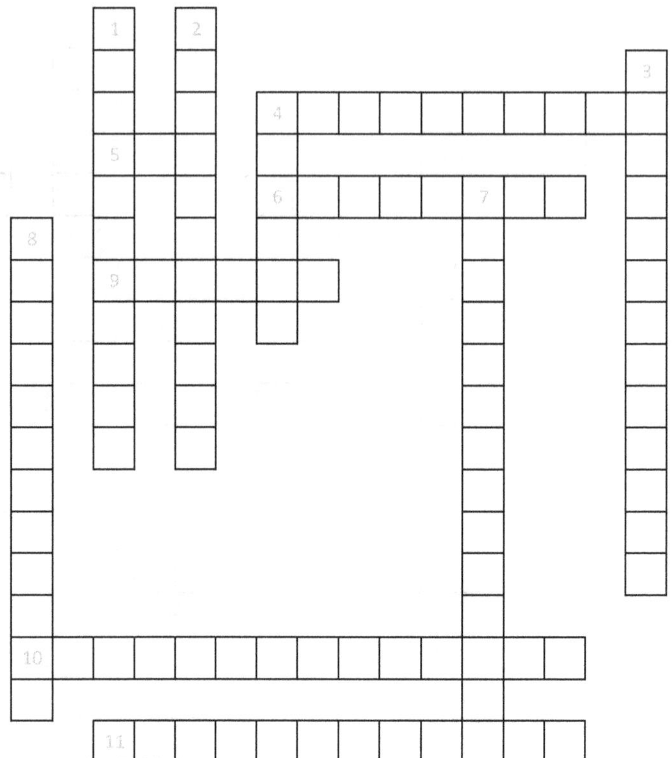

Across

4. The act of copying someone's words, ideas, results and presenting them as original content.
5. A printed, optical or electronic document designed to record all of the protocol-required information on each trial subject.
6. A written, formal clarification in an essential trial document.
9. Clinical pharmacology studies in healthy volunteers (sometimes subjects), to determine the safety, tolerability, other dynamic effects of the drug/product, and its pharmacokinetic profile.
10. Randomization scheme that changes over time depending on the data generated in a trial.
11. Compounds obtained from High Thoroughput Screening process that demonstrates the ability to interact with the desired target.

Down

1. Compounds obtained from High Throughput Screening Process.
2. US-FDA regulations on Institutional Review Boards.
3. The pieces of information in a clinical trial that have not been recorded even though they should have been collected.
4. First in man studies or trials.
7. Collection of information about each subject during the course of a trial.
8. Storage of data under proper environment and access control, after the completion of a trial.

Crossword # 94

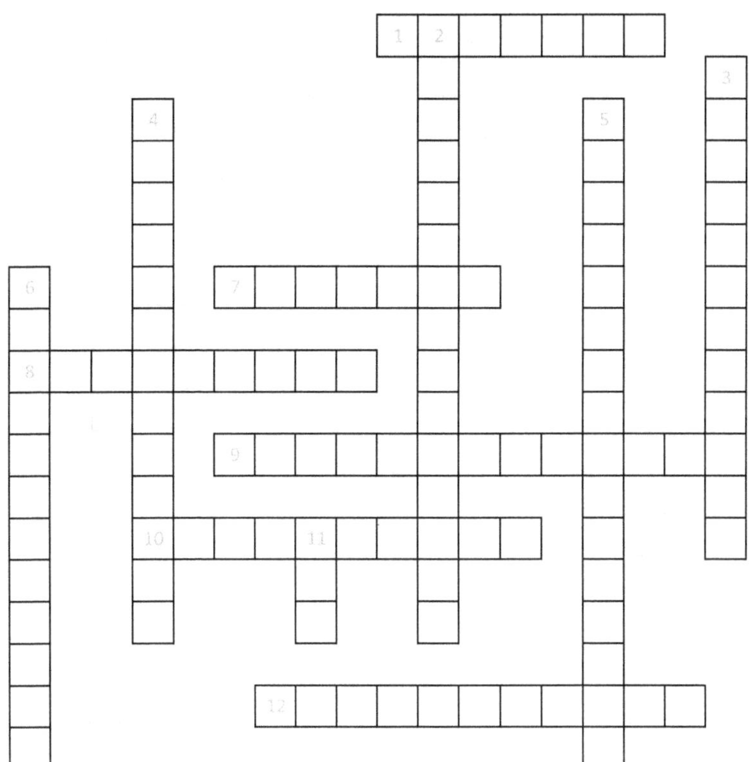

Across

1. Willful oversight in performing a particular activity.
7. Refer to Newborn baby.
8. Protocol, ICF, IB and CRF constitutes ____________ clinical trial documents.
9. Primary or secondary outcomes used to judge the effectiveness of a treatment.
10. A state in which a person is no longer able to manage his or her affairs due to physical and mental disability.
12. A contract to perform a part of or all the obligations of another contract.

Down

2. A procedure by which certain type of research, involving no more than minimal risk, may be reviewed by the chairperson of the ethics committee or designee, without convening a meeting of the entire EC.
3. An environment in which system access is controlled by persons, who are responsible for the content of electronic records.
4. A person (18 years of age and above), who is related and has maintained a regular contact with the prospective trial subject.
5. A clinical study designed to demonstrate the efficacy of a product.
6. Treatment of cancer using chemical agents.
11. Studies conducted to assess the long term safety of the approved and marketed drug/ device.

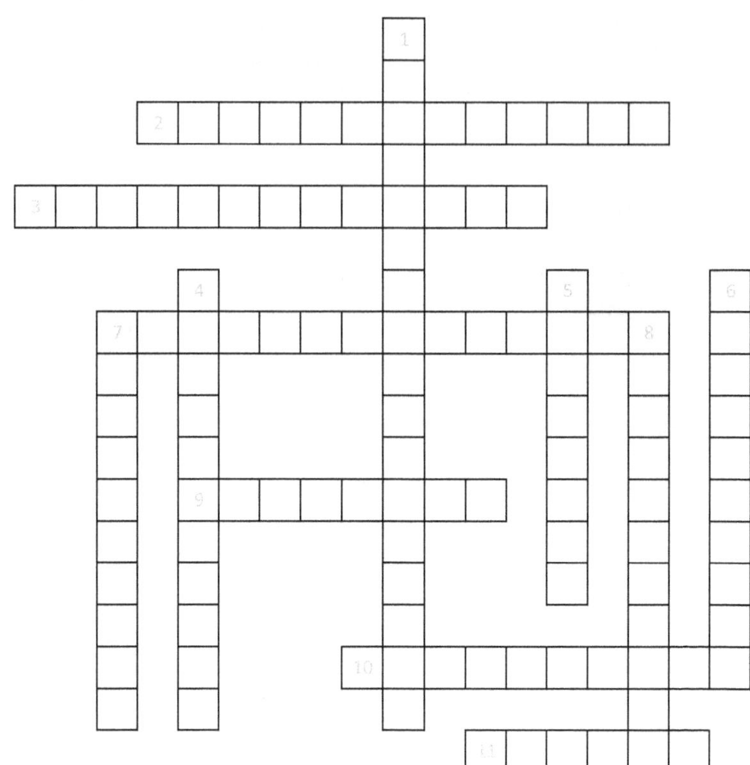

Across

2. Statistical test to determine whether there is an association between two categorical variables.
3. Refer to the subject that does not respond to the trial drug or therapy.
7. Medical management of a patient based on established regimen or guidelines.
9. Unacceptable subject recruitment involving undue inducements, duress or indirect pressure to participate in a clinical trial.
10. The act of overseeing the progress of a clinical trial, and of ensuring that it is conducted, recorded and reported in accordance with the protocol, standard operating procedure, GCP and applicable regulatory requirements.
11. The process of assigning data to categories, having a unique identifier for analysis.

Down

1. Indicator of the relative variability of a variable around its mean.
4. Recording and reporting of false data or results.
5. A dedicated area for the conduct of clinical trials, having required infrastructure and access control facilities.
6. The act of overseeing the progress of a clinical trial.
7. A person with the authority to oversee the work of a person or group.
8. Submission of documents to regulatory authorities via computer files.

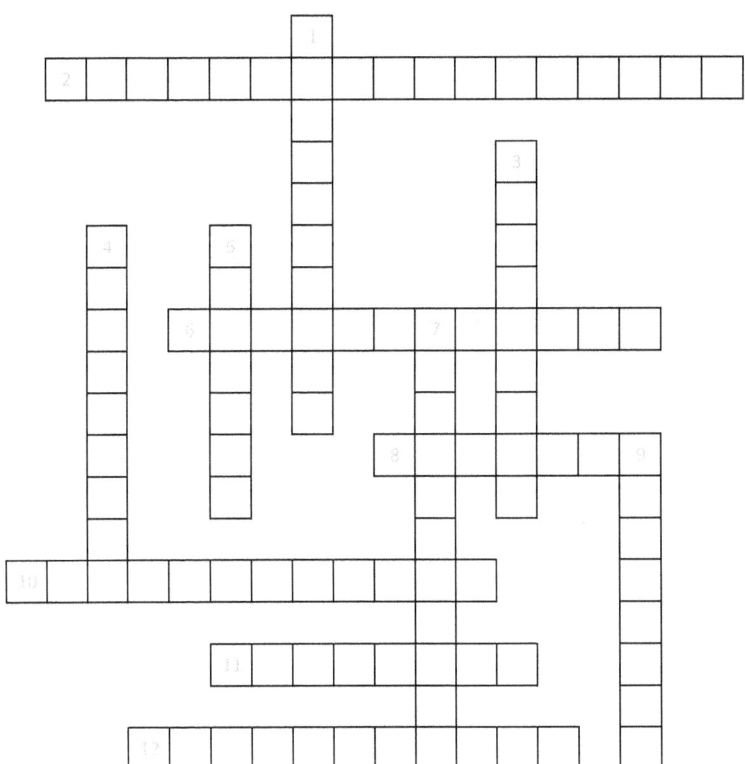

Across

2. A laboratory finding which is taken as being predictive of important clinical outcomes in the patient.
6. A set of patient numbers which are grouped together for statistical purposes.
8. A medicinal product with the same active ingredient as that of an innovator drug is known as ______________ Drug.
10. Medical care or payment provided to a subject for trial related injuries.
11. Data on important co-factors associated with a disease state ____________ Data.
12. A medical procedure that doesn't involve skin break.

Down

1. A document to demonstrate that a procedure, process and activity will consistently lead to the expected results is known as __________ Certificate.
3. A type of study in which both the investigator and subject knows which treatment the subject is receiving __________ _________ Study.
4. A display of the shape of distribution for numeric variables useful for examining a single numeric value.
5. IND application form.
7. Time frame for submitting summary report to licensing authority (DCGI) for studies discontinued prematurely.
9. A written, dated and signed agreement between two or more involved parties that sets out arrangements on delegation and distribution of tasks and financial matters.

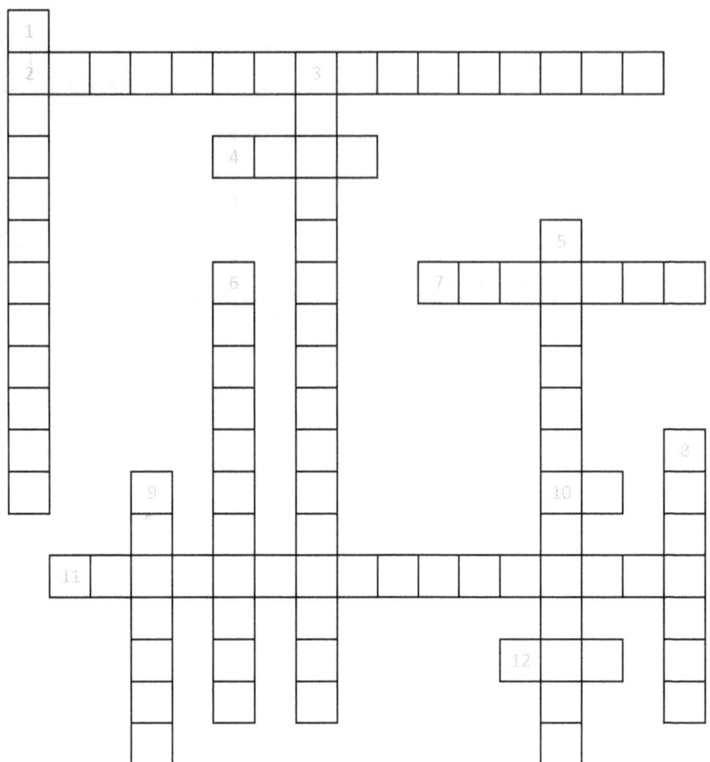

Across

2. A person who is independent of a trial, and who witness the adequacy of informed consent process, if the subject and his/her legally acceptable representative are unable to read and write.
4. Recorded information regardless of form (manual or electronic).
7. An inactive substance designed to resemble the drug being tested.
10. A document containing the details on the qualification, experience and personal details of a person.
11. A person who is independent of the trial and who witnesses the adequacy of the informed consent process if the subject and/or his/her legally acceptable representative is illiterate.
12. A person who assists the investigator in the management of a trial at a site.

Down

1. A well controlled, randomized study to evaluate the safety and efficacy of a new drug in patients with relevant disease condition.
3. The entity responsible for the pharmacological action of a drug substance.
5. A trial design in which subject is randomly assigned to receive either the standard treatment or the investigational drug.
6. US-FDA regulations on protection of human subjects.
8. Post marketing studies to collect the additional safety data from a larger patient population.
9. A device that is placed permanently into a tissue or surgically formed cavity of the human body.

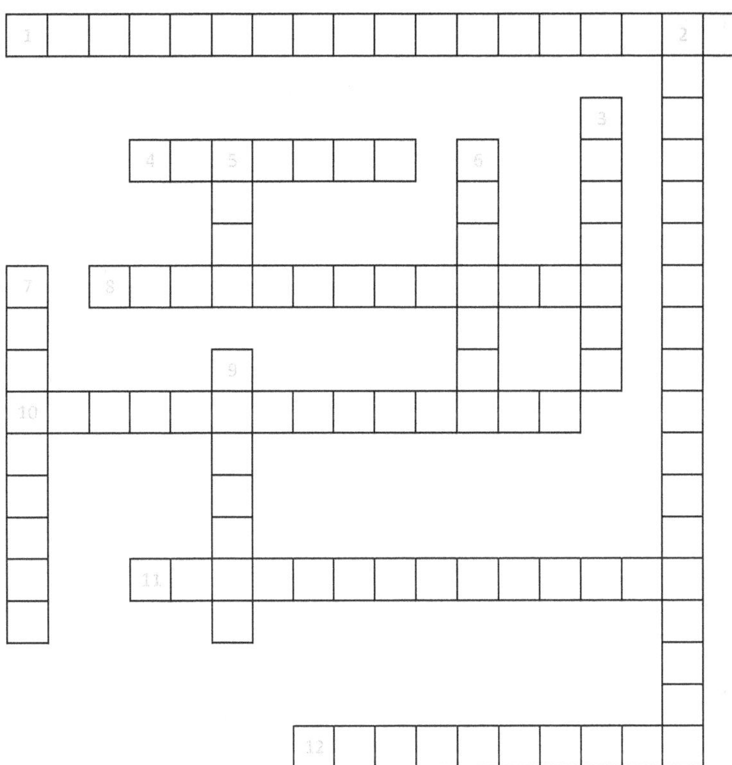

Across

1. A non- interventional study, where investigator observes the subject and interprets the outcomes.
4. A list of commitments and requirements by the FDA for each investigator performing drug/biologic studies.
8. The care provided to patients when they are admitted to a hospital or health care centre.
10. Documents narrating the conversation or discussion between two or more parties for e.g. letters, emails, fax, telephonic logs etc.
11. A process of ensuring the accuracy of a clinical trial data using manual checks, computer generated edits, reports or listings.
12. An official review of documents, facility, records and any other resources related to clinical trial by a regulatory authority at the site of the trial.

Down

2. Methods and strategy used to determine the point at which the overall study data will be considered validated.
3. Deviation from standard operating procedure(s) or the regulatory guidelines is termed as ___________ deviation.
5. Application filed to seek approval for marketing a generic drug product.
6. Means "I shall please" in Latin.
7. A particular method of performing a task.
9. A component or a substance that is analyzed employing an analytical technique.

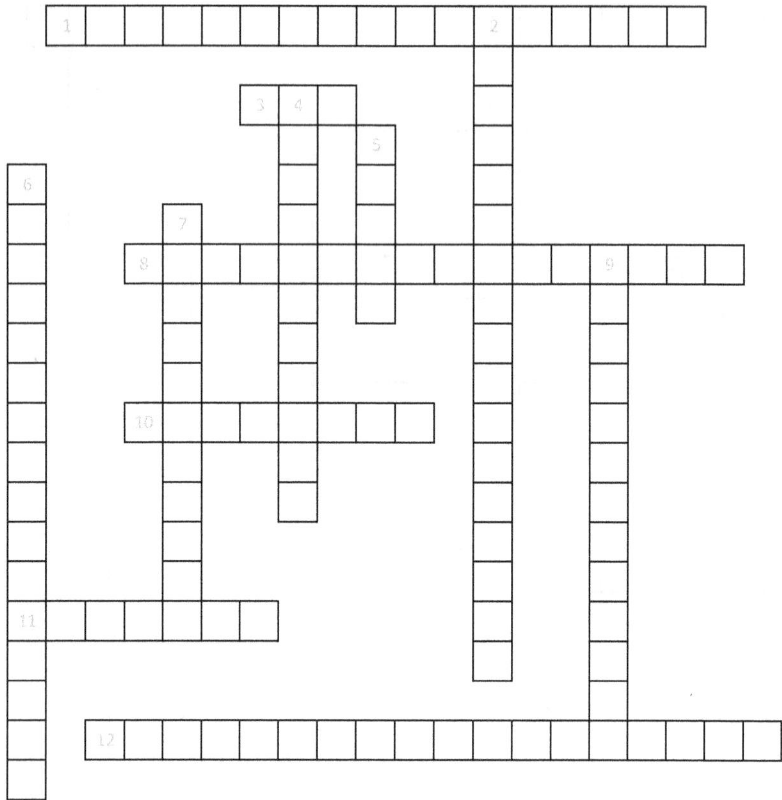

Across

1. Refers to a chemical molecule that after undergoing clinical trials could translate into a potential drug for the cure/treatment of a disease.
3. An analytical report of a batch of investigational product highlighting its content uniformity and percentage purity.
8. LD50/ED50.
10. A site visit by an FDA investigator to find out whether GCP requirements are being followed.
11. An individual who participates in a clinical trial either as a recipient of the investigational product or as a control.
12. The research in an institution that is supported by external funding.

Down

2. Extending the expiry date on the label of an investigational product.
4. The unauthorized use of a drug for an indication, which is not approved by the regulatory authorities.
5. Number of years for which IRB/IEC should retain all records after the completion of the trial.
6. A clinical trial design in which investigational product is compared with an approved drug or placebo.
7. Disaster that lead to Kefauver Harris Amendment of 1962.
9. Deviation from the protocol, standard operating procedures or applicable regulatory guidelines.

Crossword # 100

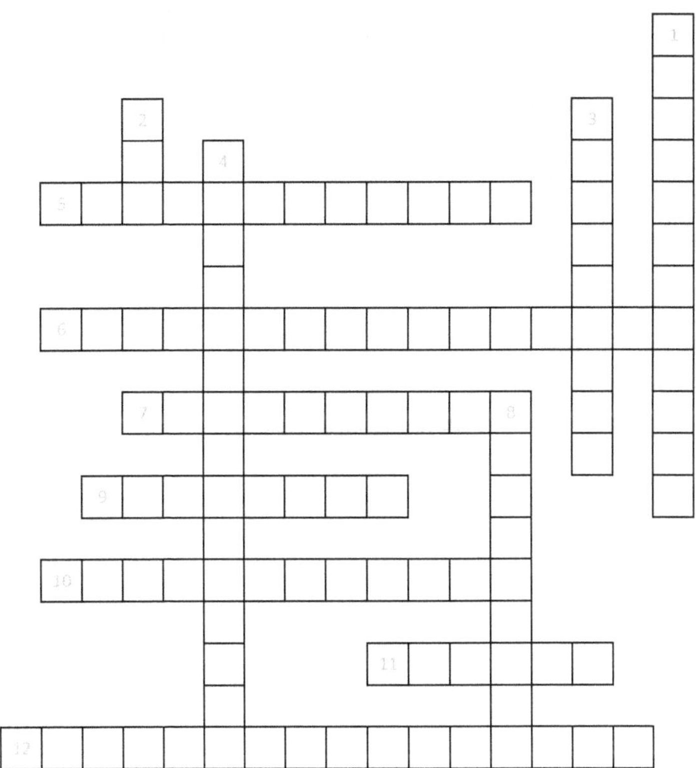

Across

5. Med Watch form for reporting safety information and adverse events to US-FDA .
6. Trials conducted to document both, therapeutic efficacy and tolerability between the generic and the original products.
7. Time frame in which an IND becomes effective if the FDA does not disapprove it.
9. Therapeutic area for which phase 1 clinical trial are conducted on patients rather than healthy volunteers.
10. A physician whose practice is not limited to a specialty is known as General ______________.
11. A document that grants the sole right of an invention to its inventor.
12. A method of providing experimental drugs/therapeutics, prior to their final regulatory approval for use in humans.

Down

1. Supervision of clinical trials by FDA.
2. Certificate of analysis is commonly denoted as __________.
3. A trial design in which all the involved parties knows the treatment group to which a subject is assigned.
4. Statistical tests used for drawing conclusions about differences between two or more groups.
8. Replacing a document with the new one after the same has been revised/ updated.

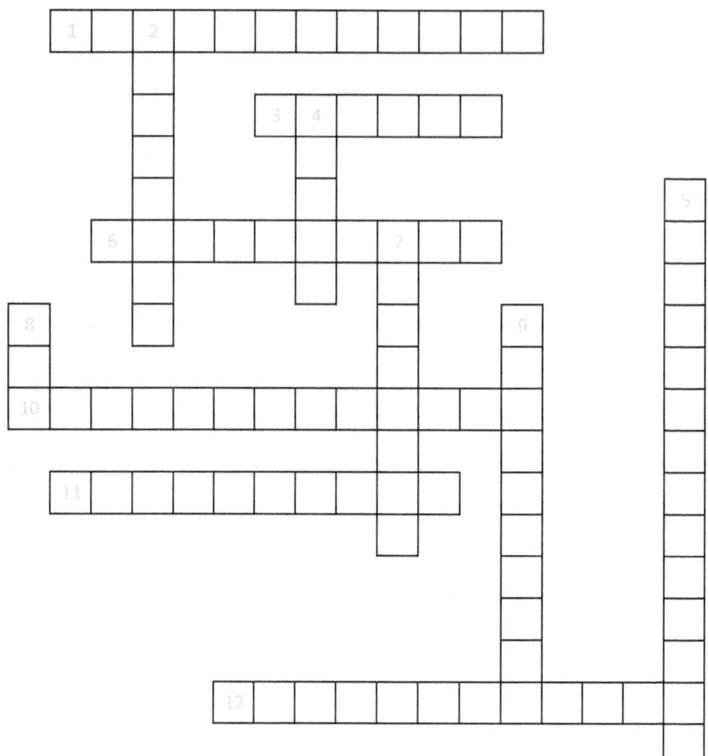

Across

1. US-FDA regulations on application for FDA approval to market a new drug.
3. Therapeutic Confirmatory Trials.
6. The process of evaluation of the hardware and software of a system, to ensure accurate and reliable compliance with user requirements.
10. Non-skilled personal care such as help with activities of daily living like bathing, dressing, eating etc.
11. An initial study to explore a new hypothesis.
12. An official communication from regulatory bodies to trial sponsor/investigator/EC documenting its decision.

Down

2. A formal written agreement which sets forth the working arrangements, between two or more parties.
4. An authorization for the use and disclosure of protected health information is known as ________________Authorization.
5. Refer to facility, equipments, personnel and processes required to carry out a clinical trial.
7. Ethical guidelines for biomedical research on human subject.
8. A person employed at a trial site for coordinating the conduct of the trial.
9. Refers to the number of people in a given population with a specific condition.

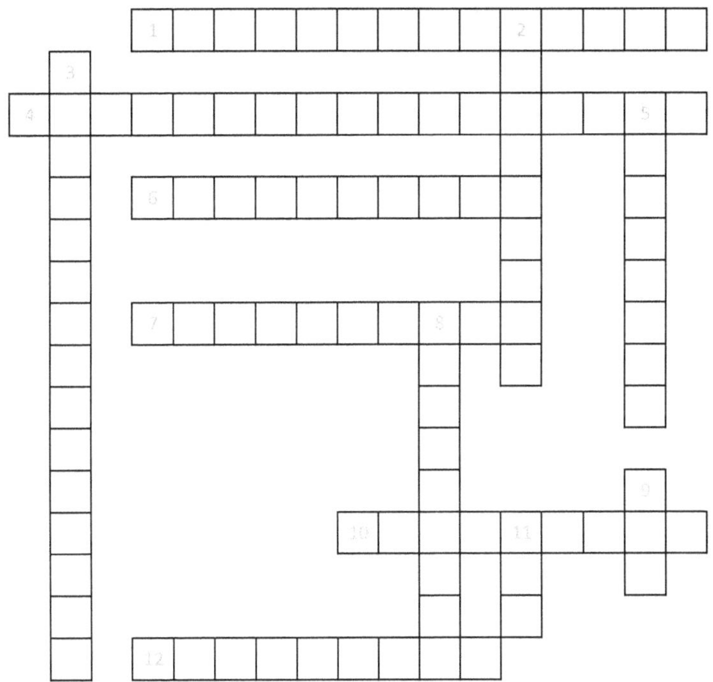

Across

1. A process of ensuring the accuracy and completeness of a clinical trial data using manual checks, computerized edits, reports or listing.
4. A novel therapy backed by strong scientific data.
6. Personnel that have been assigned specific trial related duties.
7. A clinical trial that address new methods of preventing disease is known as ___________ Trial.
10. A query generated during the data entry or review of a clinical trial data.
12. Changes made to essential trial documents (such as protocol, ICD, IB etc.) that have an impact on overall conduct of the study.

Down

2. Written description of a change(s) to protocol or formal clarification of a protocol is known as Protocol _____________.
3. A pharmaceutical form of an active ingredient or placebo being tested or used as a reference in a clinical trial including a marketed product when used in an unapproved indication or dosage form.
5. A person who is confined to custody.
8. A type of drug dosage form used for achieving immediate action.
9. Treatment groups in a randomized trial.
11. Refer to an individual's sense of general well-being and ability to perform various tasks.

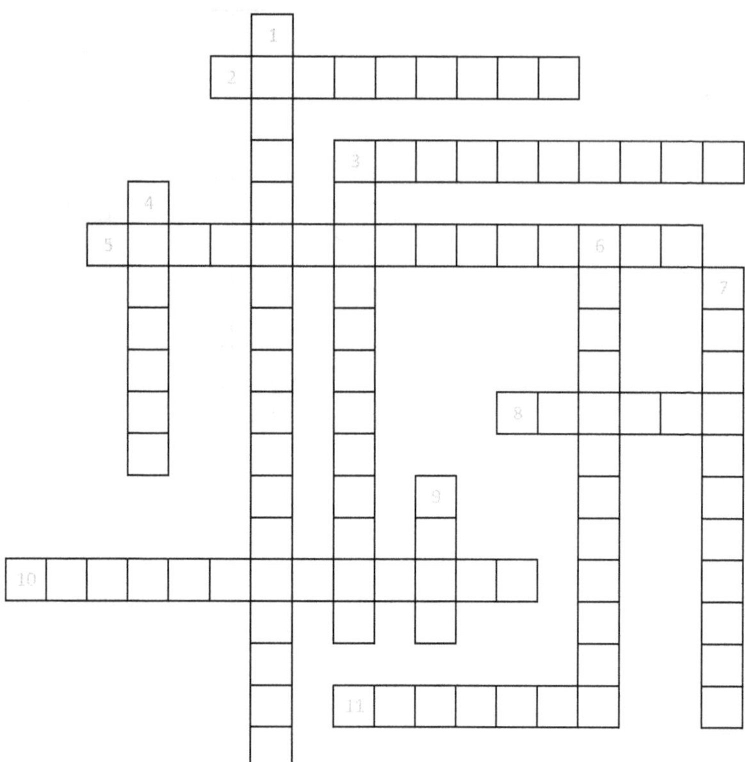

Across

2. A list of drugs and their dosages to be used in a particular health plan.
3. A systematic and independent examination of trial related activities and documents.
5. Prevention of disclosure of proprietary information to unauthorized individuals.
8. A process by which a child provides his/her willingness to participate in a clinical trial.
10. A product information sheet that summarizes all the clinical and non-clinical information of a drug product.
11. Refer to an observation that is numerically distant from rest of the data.

Down

1. Professional, personal or financial interest that can unduly bias an individual to perform his/her duties.
3. A type of non-commercial IND.
4. A report issued by FDA, following an audit that details the deficiencies requiring correction and other pertinent observations of the auditors.
6. A person who is responsible for the conduct of a clinical trial at a site.
7. ____________ Certificate is a document that captures the description and the quantity of a clinical trial material destroyed.
9. ICH topic codes.

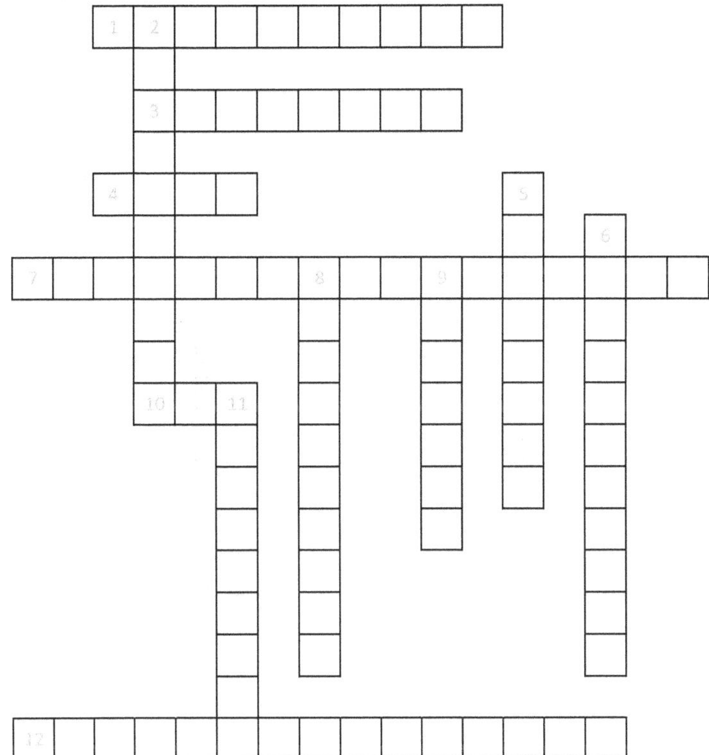

Across

1. A marketed product or placebo used as a reference in a clinical trial.
3. FDA code that represents priority review for drugs having significant advantage over existing treatments.
4. A federal government agency that issues assurances and oversees compliance of regulatory guidelines by research institutions.
7. The concentration range over which a drug has a therapeutic effect, without having unacceptable toxicity.
10. The guidelines published by FDA in the year 1997.
12. A group of trial participants having similar characteristics.

Down

2. Refers to the relocation of business processes from one country to another.
5. Number of principles in ICH-GCP Guidelines.
6. A list of commitments and requirements by the FDA, for each investigator performing drug/biologic studies.
8. The act of breaking the blinding codes of a clinical trial.
9. A process by which a subject voluntarily confirms his or her willingness to participate in a particular trial, after having been informed of all the aspects of the trial.
11. Refers to a factor that defines a system and its performance.

Crossword # 105

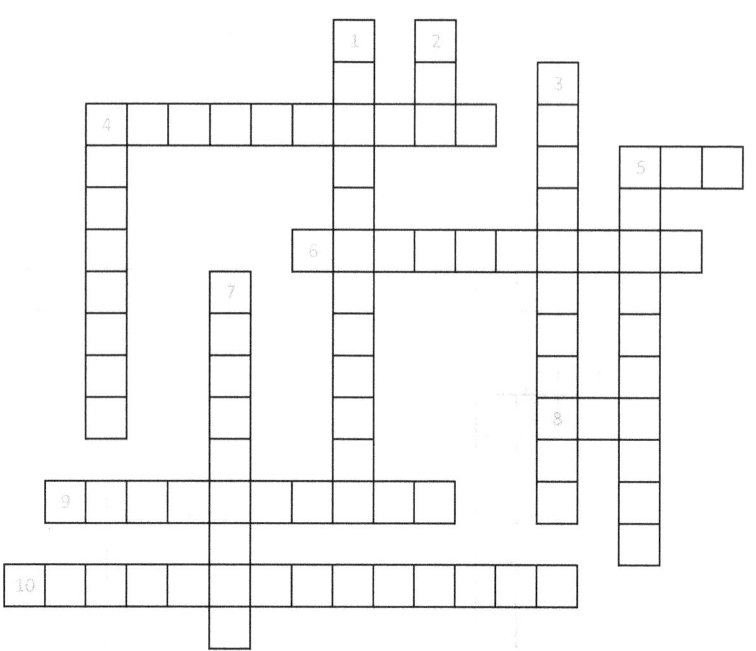

Across

4. Distribution free test that is applied when the data is not normally distributed is referred to as Non _____________ Test.
5. A person employed by a sponsor/CRO to monitor the conduct and progress of a trial.
6. An independent personnel or organization, hired for performing a specific duty.
8. Refers to legislation.
9. The scientific rationale behind a research project.
10. US-FDA regulations on reporting of IND safety reports for drugs and biologics.

Down

1. Refer to organisms of different but related species.
2. A classification of regulatory inspection outcome that requires voluntary action or response.
3. A therapy that alters the genetic structure of cells for treating genetic diseases.
4. A place where drug is prepared and dispensed.
5. An agreement between a university and corporate partners for a specific research project or program.
7. Refers to any observable characteristic or trait of an organism such as morphology, biochemical or physiological properties.

Crossword # 106

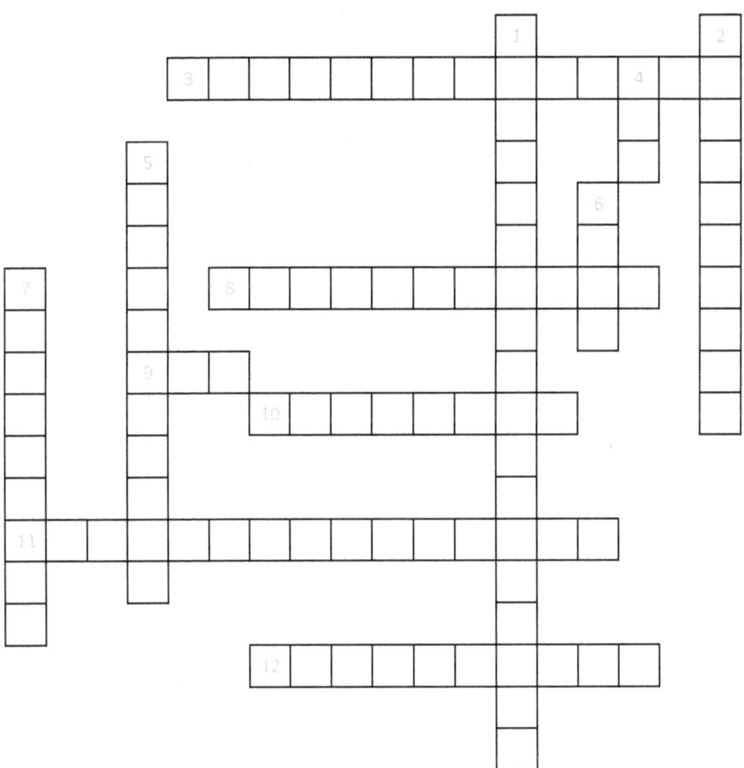

Across

3. Health service offered on outpatient basis without requiring hospitalization.
8. Most effective administration technique if the drug is required to act systematically.
9. Clinical Trial Exemption is commonly denoted as _________.
10. Storage of data/records at the end of a trial for a stipulated timeframe.
11. Document that provides public assurance for the protection of rights, safety and wellbeing of human subjects involved in a clinical trial_____________ __________ Document.
12. Text or numbers generated during the analysis of a clinical trial data.

Down

1. Investigation of the pharmacological activity of a new compound using a wide array of chemical and biochemical assays, cell culture models and animal models in a laboratory.
2. Refers to a study subject who does not complete the protocol specified visits in a clinical trial.
4. Refers to a treatment group in a randomized trial.
5. Publishing the results of a clinical trial in a peer-reviewed journal.
6. Safety reporting of marketed drugs in a specified period of time (generally on an annual basis).
7. Refer to discovery of a new drug, device, method, process or useful improvement upon any of these.

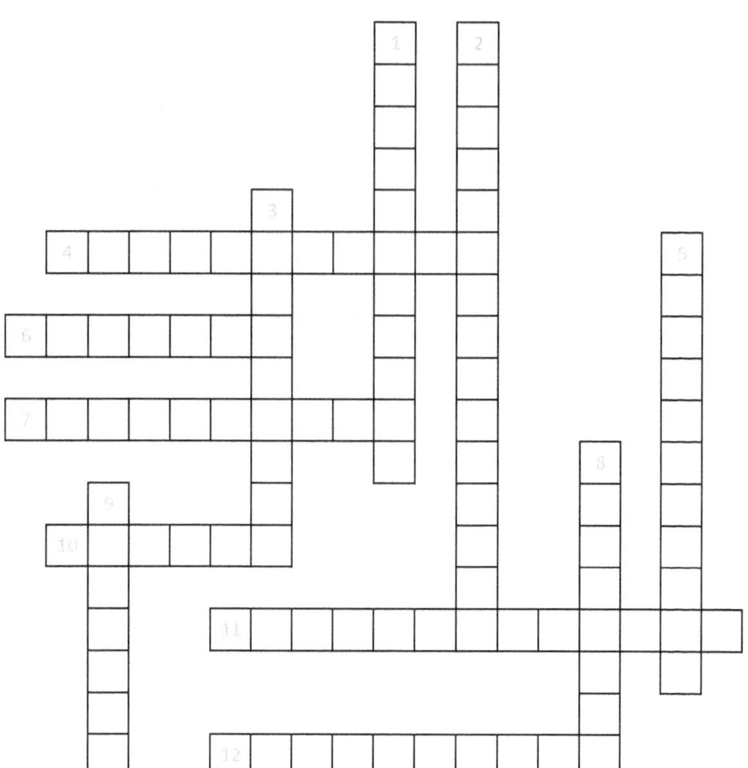

Across

4. An estimate of survivor function is known as ____________ __________Estimate.
6. A condition that impairs the normal functioning of an organism or body.
7. Allocation of specific trial related duties to the individual study team members in a clinical trial.
10. The absence of extraneous material in a drug product.
11. Refers to records that describe or document study methods, conduct and results.
12. A list of relevant published literature on a topic along with complete citation.

Down

1. The act of enrolling subjects according to the inclusion/exclusion criteria.
2. Process by which vernacular language translation of a trial document is back translated in to English.
3. Refer to the quantity of goods and materials available in the stock.
5. A measure that determines the degree to which the movement of two variables is associated is known as ________________Coefficient.
8. The process of absorption, distribution, metabolism and excretion of a drug or a vaccine in a living organism is referred to as Pharmaco_____________.
9. Dissection of a dead body to determine the cause of death and relevant medical facts.

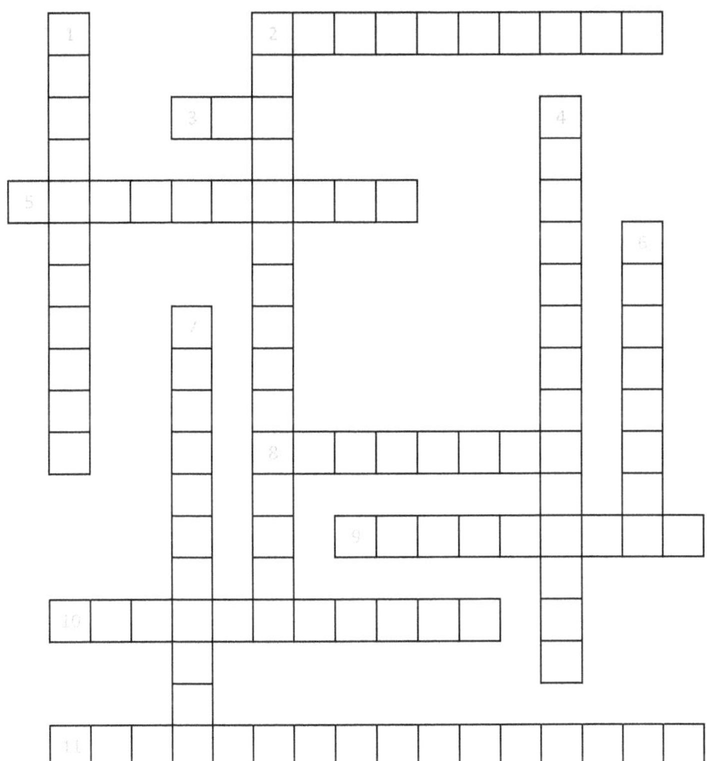

Across

2. Refers to the documentation of activities that allows reconstruction of the course of events.
3. Association responsible for developed Declaration of Helsinki.
5. A process by which compliance with essential requirements is evaluated (Assessment).
8. Refers to an individual who is legally authorized to consent on behalf of a child for participation in a clinical trial.
9. A state of physical and mental soundness.
10. A mixture of chemicals and/or biological substances and excipients for preparing a dosage form.
11. The processes of absorption, distribution, metabolism, and excretion of a drug or vaccine in a living organism.

Down

1. A type of bias that occurs when the two treatment groups that are being compared, contains different type of patients.
2. At preclinical testing the regulatory bodies generally ask for_______________ profile of drug.
4. Documents narrating the conversation or discussion between two or more parties.
6. An individual who is legally authorized to consent on behalf of a child, for participation in a clinical trial.
7. A unique identifier assigned to a clinical study for its easy identification.

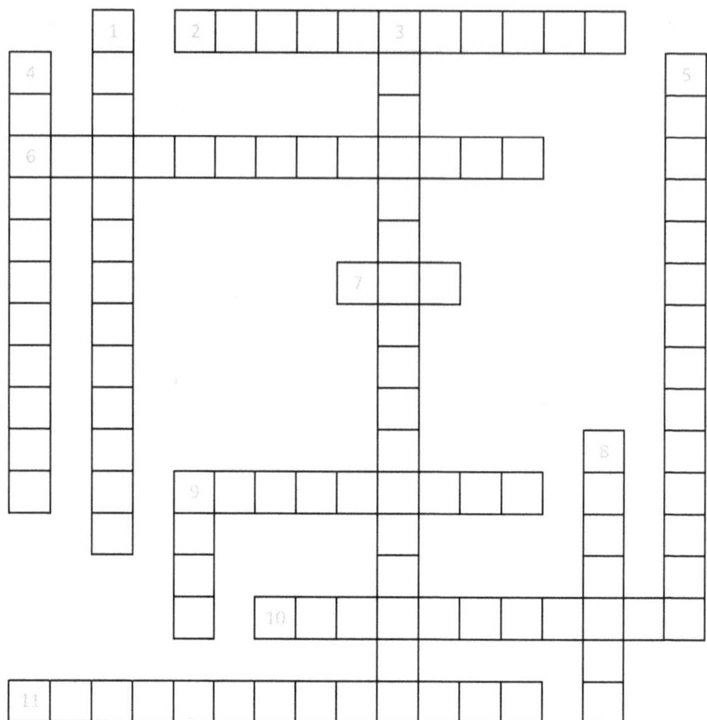

Across

2. US-FDA regulations on electronic records and electronic signatures.
6. Refers to a system of making experimental drugs available to individuals, who are unable to participate in clinical trials.
7. Ethical and scientific quality standards for designing, conducting, recording and reporting trials that involves participation of human subjects.
9. Refers to a variable that has an influence on another dependent variable.
10. Time period for which the patent of a drug is valid.
11. Refers to the variability or differences between the results of studies included in a systemic review.

Down

1. A reference book that contains official listing of marketed drugs.
3. Methods for the assessment and prevention of adverse events.
4. Needle placed in the arm with blood thinner to prevent the blood from clotting inside the needle or tubing.
5. Time frame for reporting serious, unexpected reactions (ADRs) that are not fatal or life-threatening to regulatory agencies as per ICH-GCP (no later than).
8. A coding system for adverse events that allocates each event to a body system and a diagnosis.
9. Regulatory Authority that grants the permission for conducting clinical trials in Europe.

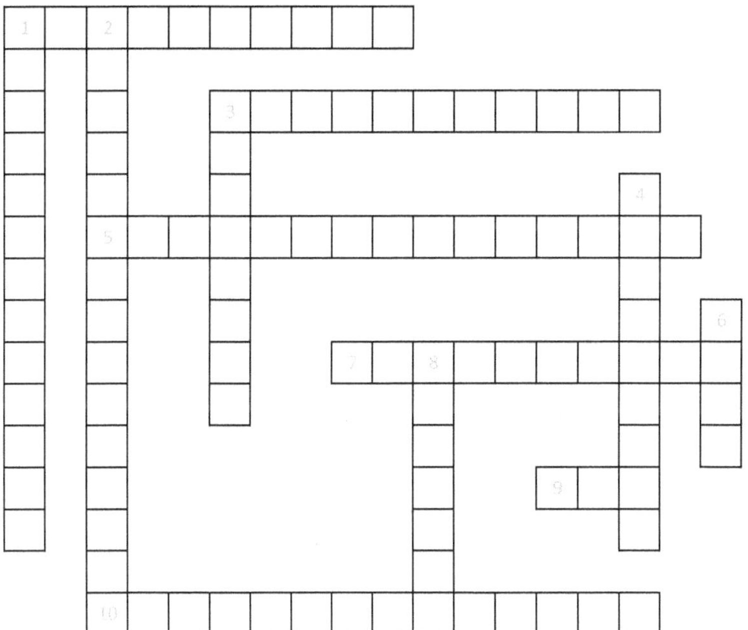

Across

1. Type-1 statistical error.
3. Analytical reports/tables for a given dataset.
5. A process by which subject voluntarily confirms his or her willingness to participate in a clinical trial.
7. Scientific rationale of a clinical trial.
9. Clinical Trial Notification is commonly denoted as _______.
10. The process, documents and records to demonstrate that IP have been used in compliance with protocol.

Down

1. Drugs that are approved by a regulatory agency to be marketed in a country.
2. ANDA packet does not include ____________.
3. Procedure for breaking the treatment codes in a blinded clinical trial.
4. Enteric coating is done to achieve the dissolution of a drug in ____________.
6. Safety reporting of marketed drugs in a specified period of time (generally on an annual basis).
8. Trials conducted after regulatory submission but prior to the drug's approval or launch.

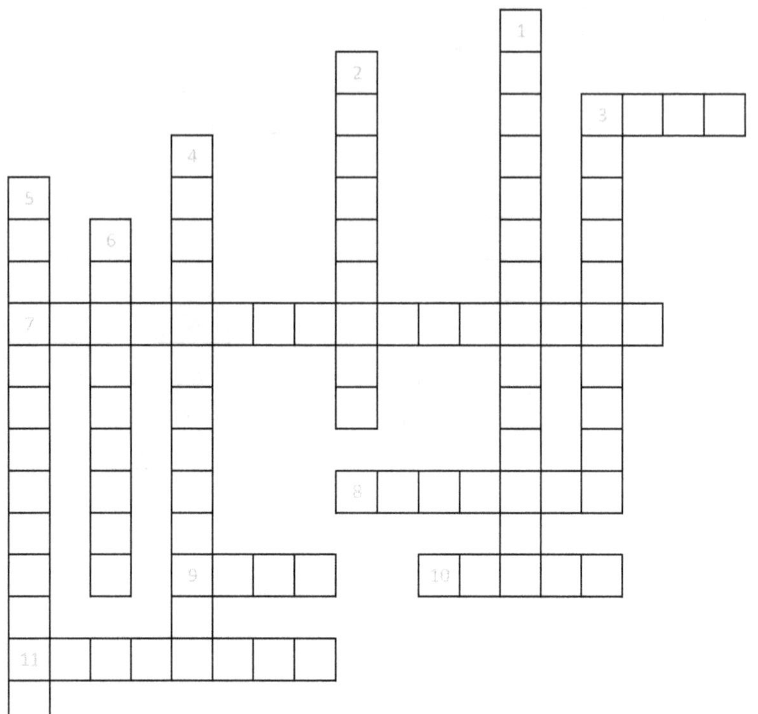

Across

3. Independent Data Monitoring Committee that may be established by the sponsor, to periodically assess the progress of a clinical trial.
7. A person who has the authority to access and review the trial related documents and activities.
8. The principle of moral rightness in action or attitude.
9. An automated interactive voice response system used to randomize or withdraw the patients in a clinical trial.
10. The difference between the smallest and largest values of a set of measurements.
11. Personal capacity to make choices, consider alternatives and act without undue influence or interference of others.

Down

1. A document that lists the core job functions of a job.
2. A new invention.
3. Refers to the release of protected health information of a study subject, by one entity to another entity.
4. The process of assigning trial subjects to treatment group using an element of chance.
5. Assays for the quantitative measurement of a drug, metabolites or chemicals in biological fluids.
6. The scientific basis or hypothesis of a clinical trial.

Crossword # 112

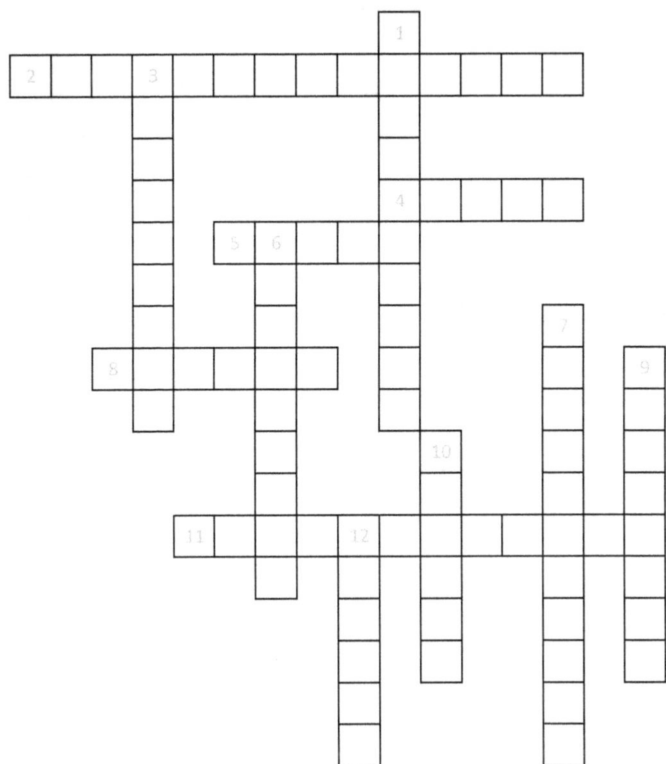

Across

2. The process whereby one determines the clinical meaning or significance of data, after the relevant statistical analysis have been performed.
4. A document for identifying a drug/placebo in compliance with applicable regulations and appropriateness of the instructions provided to the subjects.
5. One of the aims of GLP is to help reduce the incidence of ___________ positive results.
8. A process by which a child provides his/her willingness to participate in a clinical trial.
11. An extremely serious and expensive health problem that could be life threatening or may cause lifelong disability.

Down

1. Number of patients required to achieve the desired statistical significance in a clinical trial.
3. Refers to a stage of being balanced or in equilibrium.
6. De-identified information of a trial participant that in no way can disclose his/her identity.
7. A therapy that alters the genetic structure of cells for treating genetic diseases.
9. A product's ability to produce beneficial effect on the course or duration of a disease.
10. The absence of extraneous material in a drug product.
12. Sequence of instructions that are interpreted or carried out by another program.

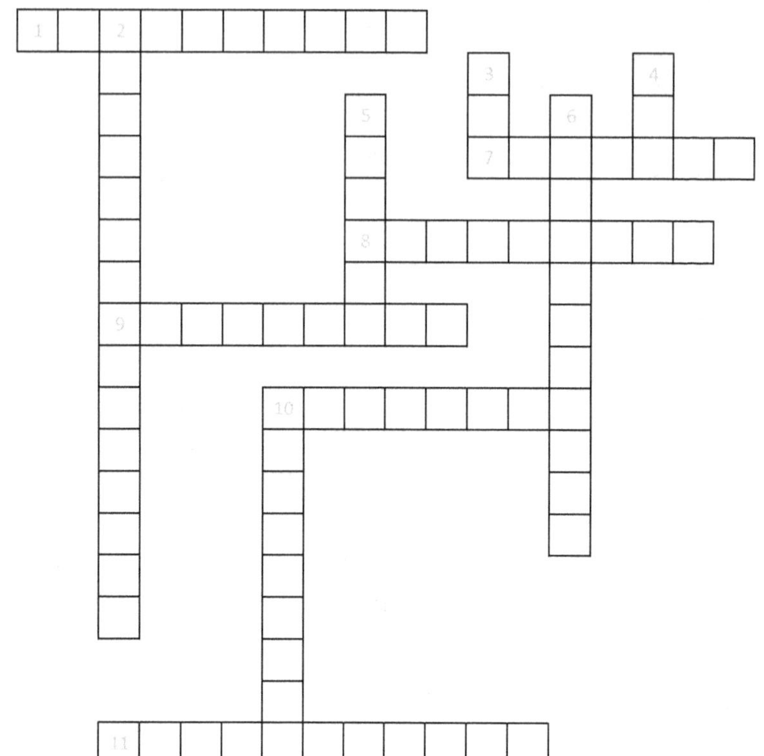

Across

1. Complexation influences ____________ of a drug.
7. Preclinical testing is mainly done on __________.
8. Non compliance to either protocol schedule of events or standard operating procedures.
9. An investigational product or marketed product or placebo used in a clinical trial.
10. A person who is confined to custody.
11. A measure of the strength of the relationship between two variables.

Down

2. The initial visit to investigator site by the Sponsor/CRO personnel for evaluating the suitability of investigator and facility.
3. Association responsible for developed Declaration of Helsinki.
4. An analytical report of a batch of investigational product highlighting its content uniformity and percentage purity.
5. A supplier of goods or services.
6. Drugs that have immediate authorization and can be sold in a country.
10. A particular method of performing a task.

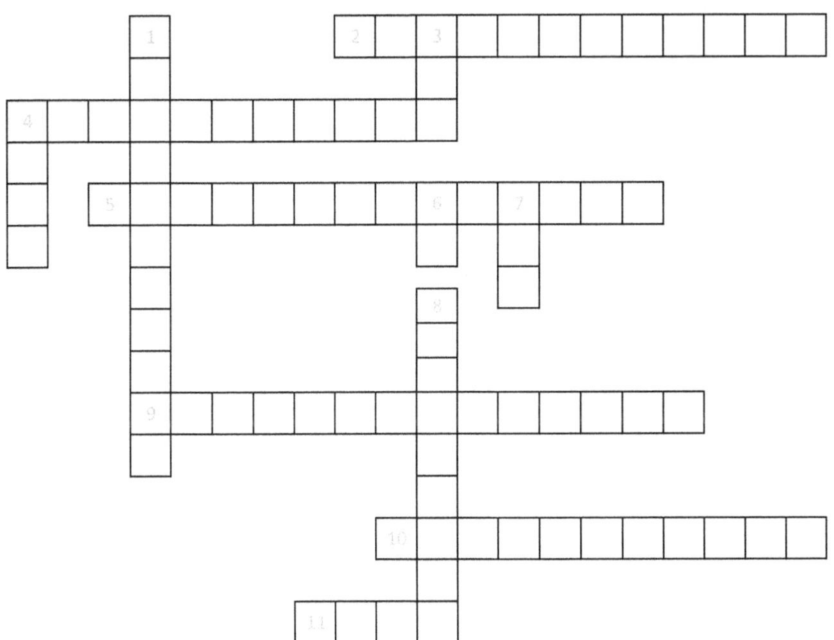

Across

2. Treatment of cancer using chemical agents.
4. US-FDA regulations on protection of human subjects.
5. Collection of information about each subject during the course of a trial.
9. Medical management of a patient based on established regimen or guidelines.
10. Recording and reporting of false data or results.
11. Most frequently occurring value in a set of data.

Down

1. The unauthorized use of a drug for an indication, which is not approved by the regulatory authorities.
3. Guidelines for the choice of control group and related issue in clinical trials.
4. The year in which Declaration of Helsinki was last amended.
6. A specific circumstance when the use of certain treatments could be harmful.
7. Regulatory Agency in Australia.
8. Term used for a potential drug substance.

Crossword # 115

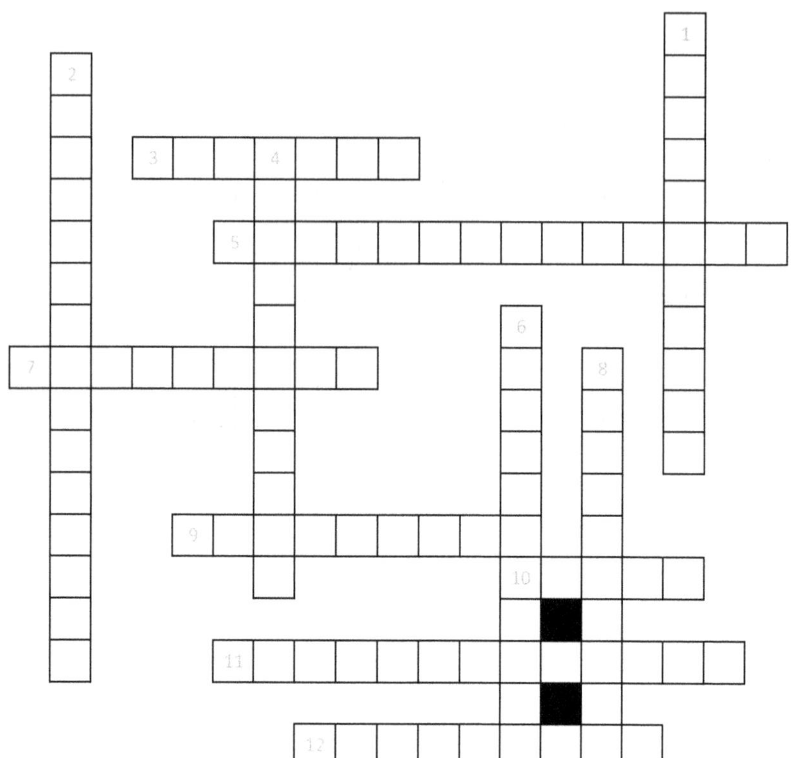

Across

3. The responsibility for the creation of essential trial documents like Protocol, ICF, and IB etc. lies with ________.
5. Health service offered on outpatient basis without requiring hospitalization.
7. A state of physical and mental soundness.
9. Errors in either collection or recording of clinical trial data.
10. Any departure of the result from the "true" value is termed as ______________.
11. A mechanism by which the access to clinical trial facility or documents is restricted to authorized individuals.
12. Refer to the quantity of goods and materials available in the stock.

Down

1. The extent of harm or discomfort anticipated from a clinical trial which is not greater than the routine practice.
2. A drug development approach that involves choosing a disease or biological target (such as enzyme, receptor, ion channel etc.) to treat and then developing a model for that disease.
4. Quantitative data such as number of patients, number of visits etc.
6. A written evaluation of the audit results by the auditor.
8. A marketed product or placebo used as a reference in a clinical trial.

Crossword # 116

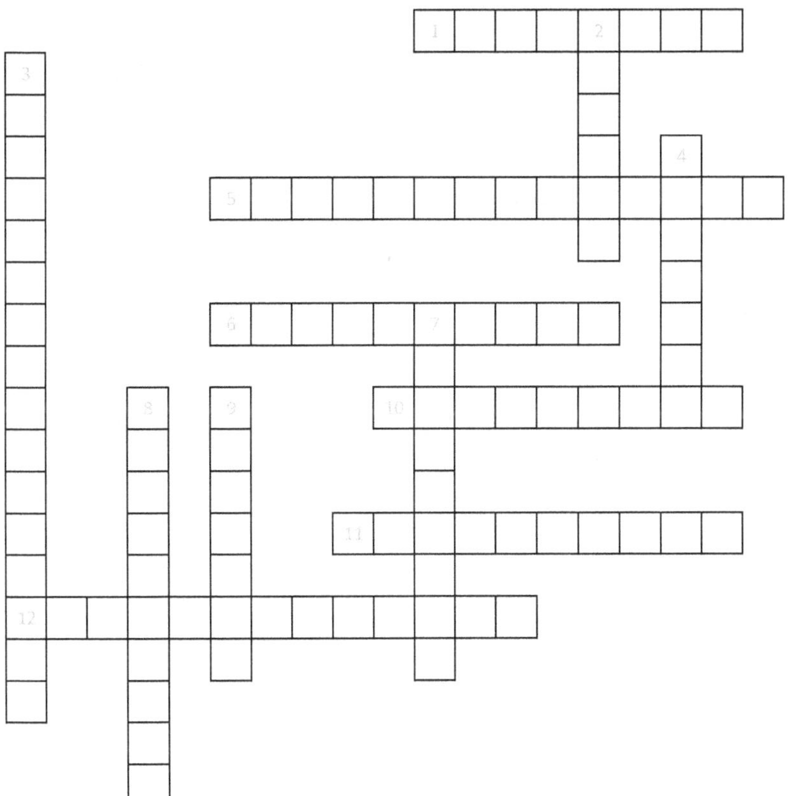

Across

1. Number of principles in ICH-GCP Guidelines.
5. Randomization scheme that changes over time depending on the data generated in a trial.
6. Forms/documents containing study specific information, required to be filled in by the study subjects.
10. A strategy employed in clinical trials comparing two treatments, where each patient receives both the treatments, one followed by other.
11. Time frame in which an IND becomes effective if the FDA does not disapprove it.
12. A document used for subject recruitment after obtaining EC approval that contains non-coercive trial information.

Down

2. Convenient and commonest drug dosage form.
3. Trials conducted to document both, therapeutic efficacy and tolerability between the generic and the original products.
4. Official or legal permission to an individual or organization by a competent authority to engage in a practice, occupation or activity.
7. A person who provides social, emotional, medical and financial support to an individual.
8. Type-1 statistical error.
9. A pre-set standard for measuring the outcome.

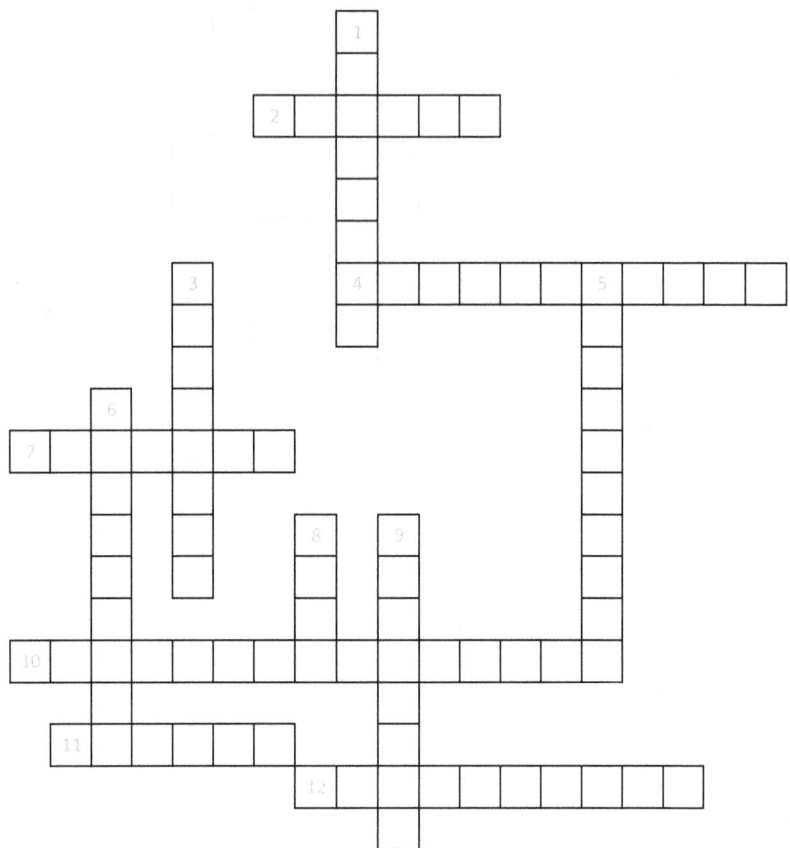

Across

2. Tests conducted inside the body of a living organism.
4. A designation of the FDA to indicate a therapy developed to treat a rare disease.
7. Respect for person, beneficence, justice are the three principles discussed in the ____________ Report.
10. Statistical analysis of trial data at a predefined time interval before all subjects has completed the trial.
11. Early stages of a developing organism (from conception to 8th week of pregnancy).
12. Personnel that have been assigned specific trial related duties.

Down

1. An amendment in the existing documents or processes.
3. Subsequent contact with a subject in order to assess current status of a subject's condition or outcome of an adverse event.
5. Refers to a study subject who does not complete the protocol specified visits in a clinical trial.
6. A step by step procedure for making a series of choice, among alternative decision to reach an outcome.
8. Recorded information regardless of form (manual or electronic).
9. An electronic platform that contains the data generated from a clinical trial.

Crossword # 118

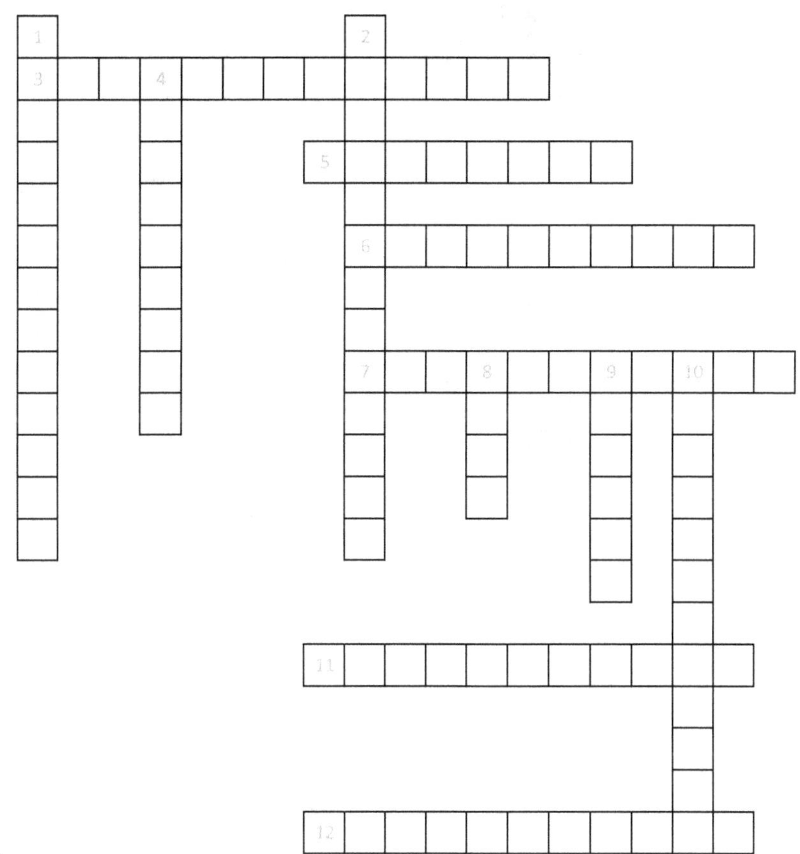

Across

3. Permission to use and share a subject's protected health information for the purpose of a research study.
5. A dedicated area for the conduct of clinical trials, having required infrastructure and access control facilities.
6. An agreement between a university and corporate partners for a specific research project or program.
7. Methodology used to investigate a drug or device for its safety and efficacy.
11. A designation of the US-FDA to indicate a therapy developed to treat a rare disease.
12. Time period for which the patent of a drug is valid.

Down

1. Refers to a system of making experimental drugs available to individuals, who are unable to participate in clinical trials.
2. A study in which a particular type of subject is equally represented in each study group.
4. A condition of being confined to home and requiring considerable efforts and assistance to leave the home.
8. Regulatory Authority responsible for regulating clinical trials in India.
9. Conforming to an accepted standard of human behavior.

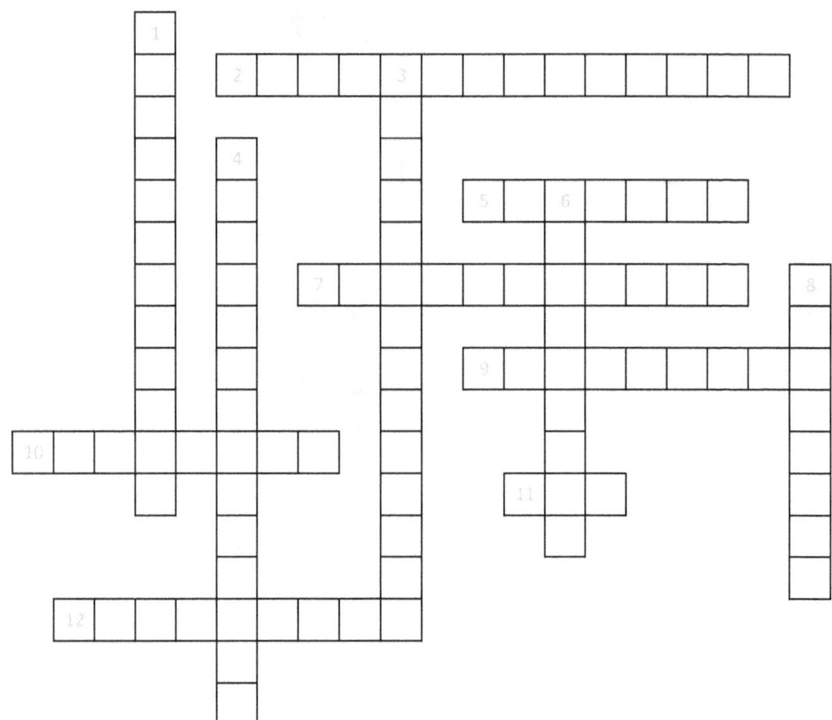

Across

2. A medically qualified personnel in an organization who supports the marketing and/ or research department.
5. Dissection of a dead body to determine the cause of death and relevant medical facts.
7. A variable that is based on categorical data and cannot be measured numerically.
9. Written description of a change(s) to protocol or formal clarification of a protocol is known as protocol ____________.
10. Federal Food and Drug Act in 1906 brought truth in ___________.
11. A person employed at a trial site for coordinating the conduct of the trial.
12. A person who submits a trial application to a regulatory agency.

Down

1. An environment in which system access is controlled by persons, who are responsible for the content of electronic records.
3. A process of providing the health care services to an individual.
4. The process of verifying the data entered in the case report form against the source data in order to establish its accuracy and completeness.
6. A name, word, symbol or phrase used to identify a particular product.
8. Personal capacity to make choices, consider alternatives and act without undue influence or interference of others.

Crossword # 120

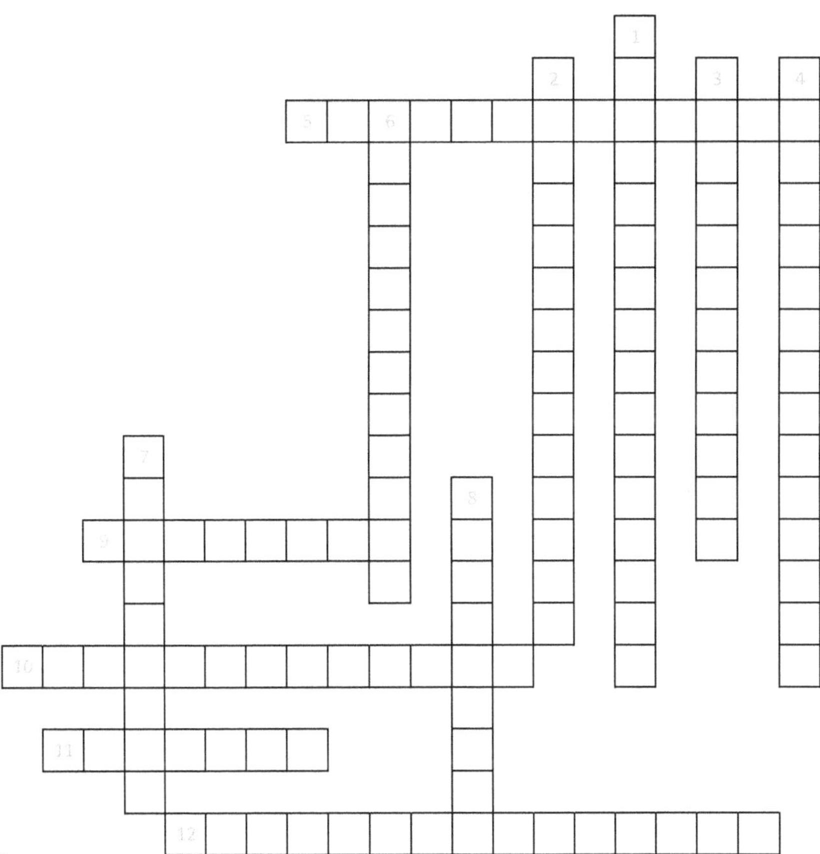

Across

5. Refers to records that describe or document study methods, conduct and results.
9. Storage of data/records at the end of a trial for a stipulated timeframe.
10. A comparison of case report form and ancillary data to the raw data in the clinical trial reporting database for the purpose of demonstrating the accuracy of data processing.
11. The number assigned to an essential document in use.
12. Official daily publication for rules, proposed rules and notices of federal agencies and organization in United States.

Down

1. Study of genetic variation underlying differential response to drugs.
2. Refer to facility, equipments, personnel and processes required to carry out a clinical trial.
3. An environment in which the access to trial related information is not controlled.
4. A type of non-commercial Investigational New Drug Application submitted by a physician who both initiates and conducts an investigation and under whose immediate direction the investigational drug is administered or dispensed.
6. The decision of regulatory authorities to put a clinical study on hold.
7. A list of drugs and their dosages to be used in a particular health plan.
8. Type-2 statistical error.

Crossword # 121

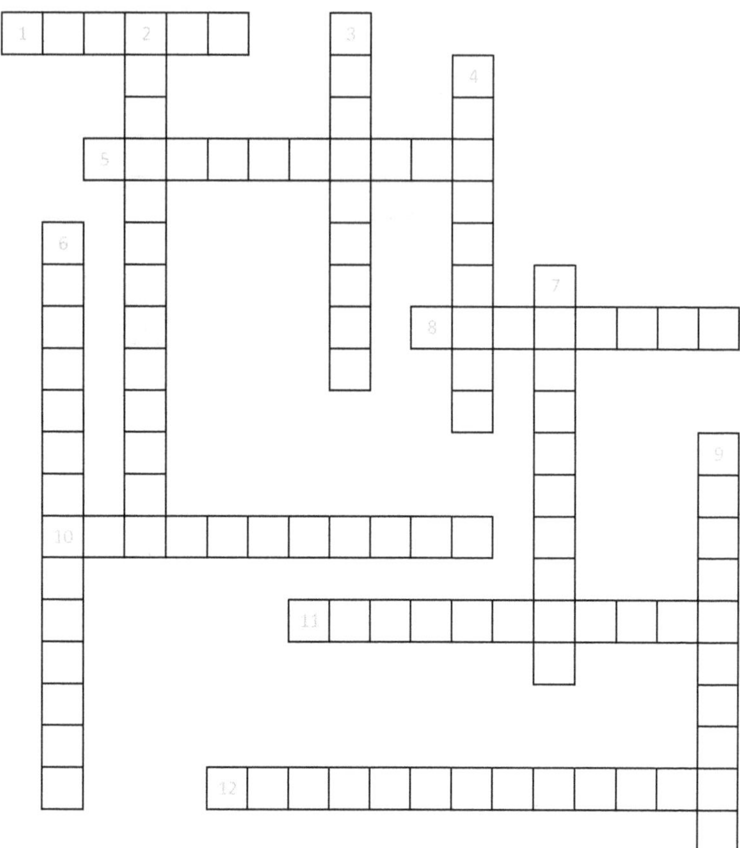

Across

1. Written instructions or rules to achieve uniformity, consistency and decision making.
5. A government order with the force of the law.
8. Measurements taken usually at the beginning of a study to serve as a reference for subsequent measurements.
10. Compounds obtained from High Throughput Screening Process.
11. A dosage form that contains one or more drug substances.
12. The process of assigning trial subjects to treatment group using an element of chance.

Down

2. Report prepared after interim analysis of data.
3. A display of the shape of distribution for numeric variables useful for examining a single numeric value.
4. Term used for a potential drug substance.
6. The information on overall general health, past illnesses and current medical problems of a subject.
7. Allocation of specific trial related duties to the individual study team members in a clinical trial.
9. Review of facility and resources are the critical elements of clinical trial __________________.

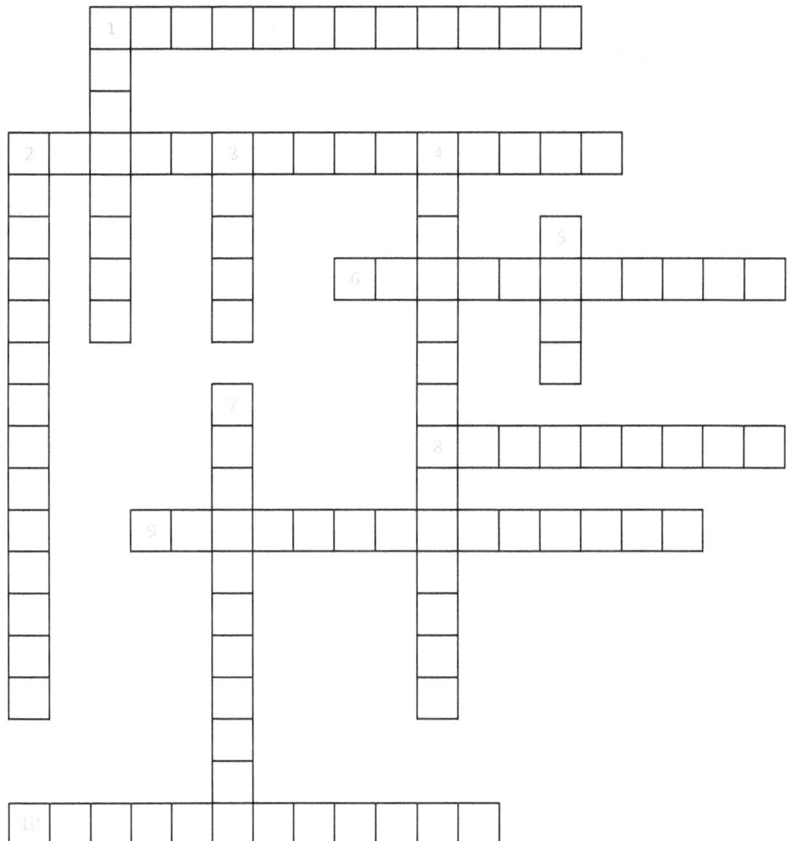

Across
1. Medical care or payment provided to a subject for trial related injuries.
2. Prevention of disclosure of proprietary information to unauthorized individuals.
6. Ownership of sole rights of a document, process or product.
8. A formal written, binding commitment.
9. A process of ensuring the accuracy and completeness of a clinical trial data using manual checks, computerized edits, reports or listing.
10. Combining the results of several studies that address a set of related research hypothesis.

Down
1. Testing in human beings is known as __________ testing.
2. Documents narrating the conversation or discussion between two or more parties.
3. Articles (other than food), intended for use in the diagnosis, cure, mitigation, treatment or prevention of disease in man or other animals.
4. The process, documents and records to demonstrate that IP have been used in compliance with protocol.
5. Facility for conducting clinical trials.
7. Any public or private entity or medical or dental facility where clinical trials are conducted.

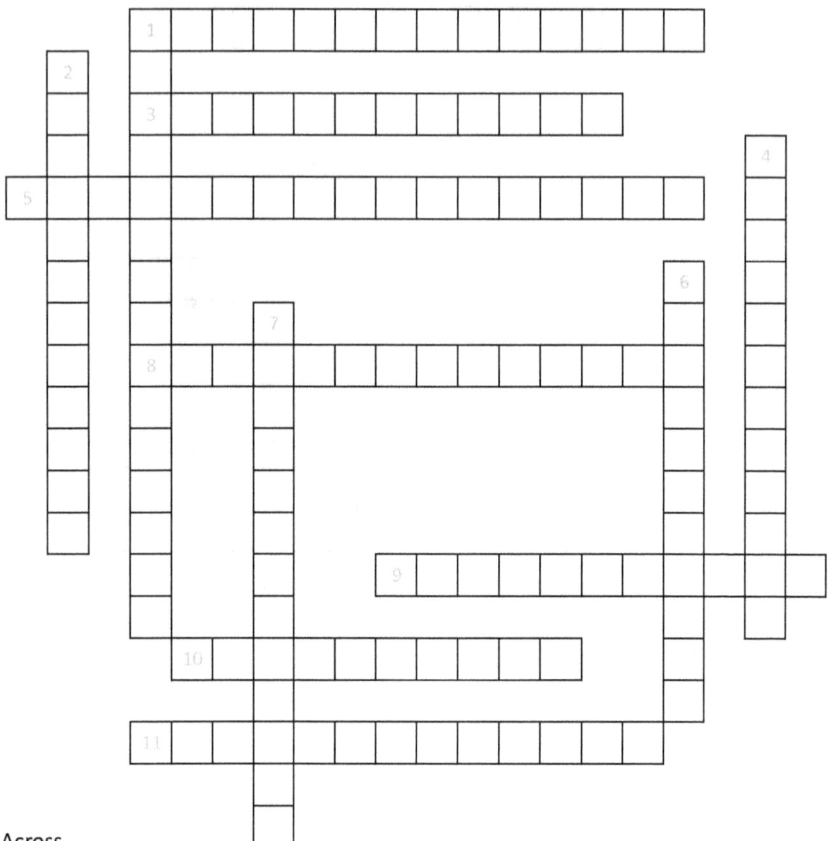

Across

1. Information systems for analysis of genomic data.
3. Data to represent situations where the event of interest (e.g. survival, death, response etc.) is not recorded for a patient.
5. Use of available published data as a control arm.
8. A patient, who does not meet the inclusion criteria, falls under the category of ________.
9. A mixture of chemicals and/or biological substances and excipients for preparing a dosage form.
10. An archival media on which essential trial documents can be transferred at a very small size.
11. Number of new events in a population during a specified period of time.

Down

1. Process by which vernacular language translation of a trial document is back translated in to english.
2. The act of making changes or amendments to an information, document or process.
4. A log that captures the dates of enrolment and other protocol required visits of a clinical trial subject.
6. Complete records of patient's disease history entered in hospital files, out-patient charts or medical records.
7. ___________study is based on historical data already existing in the records.

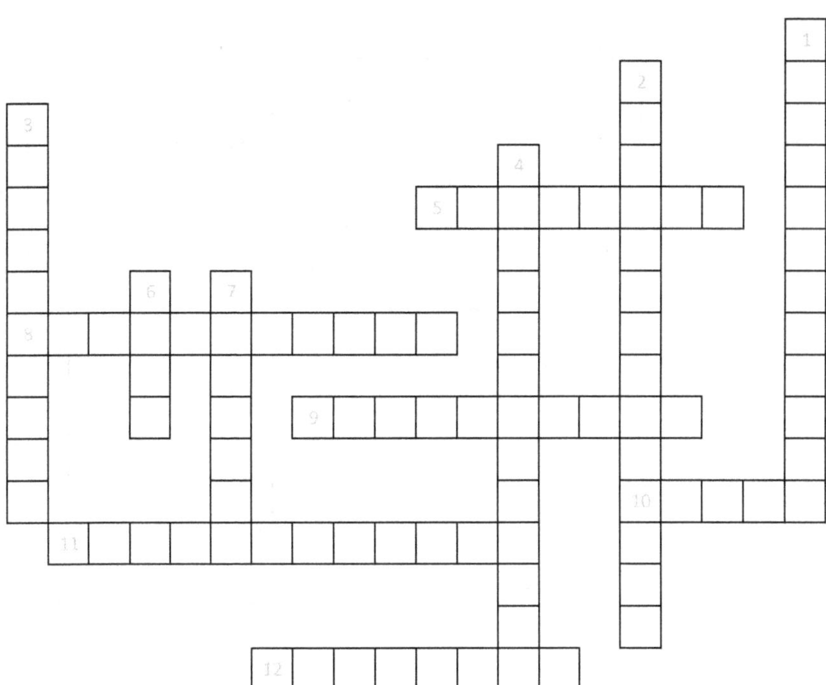

Across

5. An individual who is legally authorized to consent on behalf of a child, for participation in a clinical trial.
8. ___________ statement is signed by investigator(s) at the end of the trial to document their compliance with ICH-GCP and applicable regulatory requirements.
9. Statistical Analysis is a part of clinical data ___________ process.
10. A person authorized to act on behalf of another person.
11. Display of relation between two numeric variables while distinguishing between levels of categorical variables.
12. A type of statistical chart that displays information about the distribution of numeric variable.

Down

1. The branch of medical science that deals with the study of incidence, distribution and control of a disease in a population.
2. A plan laid to define the monitoring visit intervals, source data verification requirements, protocol specifying monitoring instructions (if any) and other elements.
3. A state in which a person is no longer able to manage his or her affairs due to physical and mental disability.
4. A product information sheet that summarizes all the clinical and non-clinical information of a drug product.
6. A Factor, element, or course of action involving an uncertain, potentially negative outcome.
7. A device that is placed permanently into a tissue or surgically formed cavity of the human body.

Across

1. Articles published in peer-reviewed scientific journals.
5. A person who has the authority to access and review the trial related documents and activities.
7. A comparison group of study subjects in a trial, who are not treated with the investigational agent.
10. A brief summary including the objectives, methods, results and conclusion of a clinical trial or any other research work.
11. A group of trial participants having similar characteristics.
12. A medically qualified personnel employed by trial Sponsor/CROs for reviewing critical medical data (safety and efficacy) of a clinical trial.

Down

2. The absence of viable, contaminating microorganisms.
3. Title 21 of the CFR, Section 312 covers __________.
4. ANDA packet does not include _____________.
6. An Individual or juridical or other body authorized under applicable law to consent on behalf of a prospective subject for participation in a clinical trial.
8. A systematic and Independent examination of trial related activities and documents.
9. Minimal concentration level at which a drug is able to produce an effect in human body is called minimum ___________ dose.

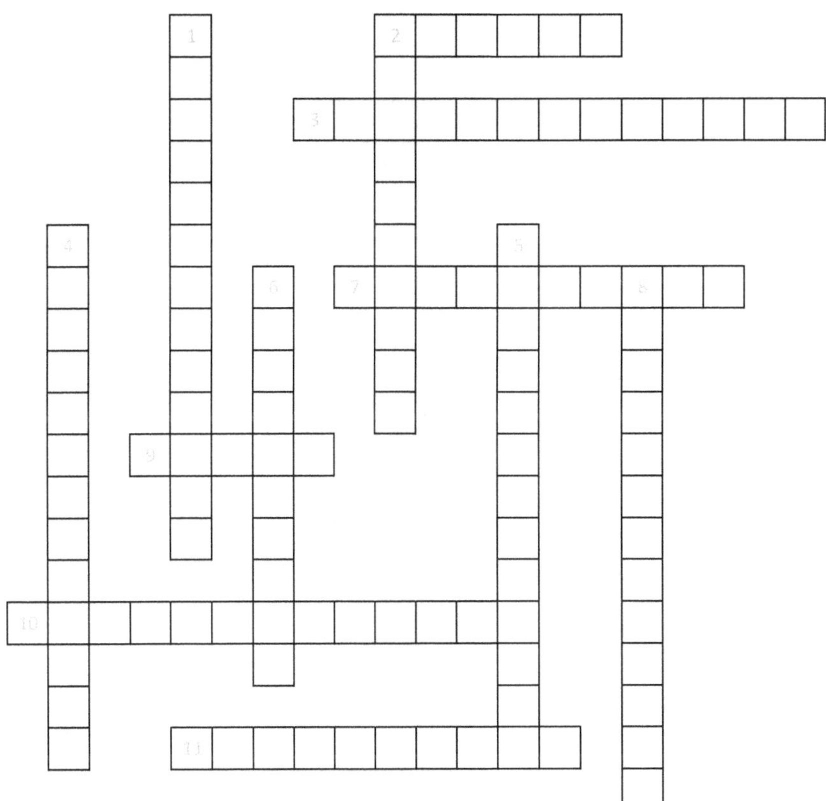

Across

2. Investigational New Drug Application is filed to initiate the testing of a drug in ______________.
3. The pieces of information in a clinical trial that have not been recorded even though they should have been collected.
7. Large scale clinical trials having a sample size of 10,000 or more that evaluates the marginally effective investigational product.
9. The physical abnormalities that are linked to an adverse event.
10. A clinical trial database in which all the validation queries have been resolved and which is ready for analysis.
11. A process by which compliance with essential requirements is evaluated (Assessment).

Down

1. Refers to the variability or differences between the results of studies included in a systemic review.
2. The scientific rationale behind a research project.
4. Technique that uses living organisms, or substances from organism, biological systems, or processes to make or modify a product or process, to change plants or animals, or to develop micro-organisms for specific uses.
5. Closing a clinical study after the same has been completed or prematurely terminated/suspended.
6. An organizational chart that describes different functional positions in an organization.
8. Yearly summary reports submitted to EC or regulatory agencies on the progress of a trial.

Across

2. Accelerated approval is also known as Accelerated ___________.
3. Action letter from the regulatory agency after review of a NDA, which signals that the drug can be approved.
5. ___________ Intervals represents a plausible range for the population value results from the sample.
7. The act of overseeing the progress of a clinical trial, and of ensuring that it is conducted, recorded and reported in accordance with the protocol, standard operating procedure, GCP and applicable regulatory requirements.
10. Indicator of the relative variability of a variable around its mean.
12. Discovery by chance.

Down

1. Scientific rationale of a clinical trial.
4. Analysis that combines the results of several studies to address a set of related research hypotheses.
6. Deviation from the protocol, standard operating procedures or applicable regulatory guidelines.
8. Drug Technical Advisory Board is the highest ___________ body, under Drug and Cosmetic Act 1940.
9. Refers to a factor that defines a system and its performance.
11. The paper used in Case Report Form (CRF) for manual entry.

Crossword # 128

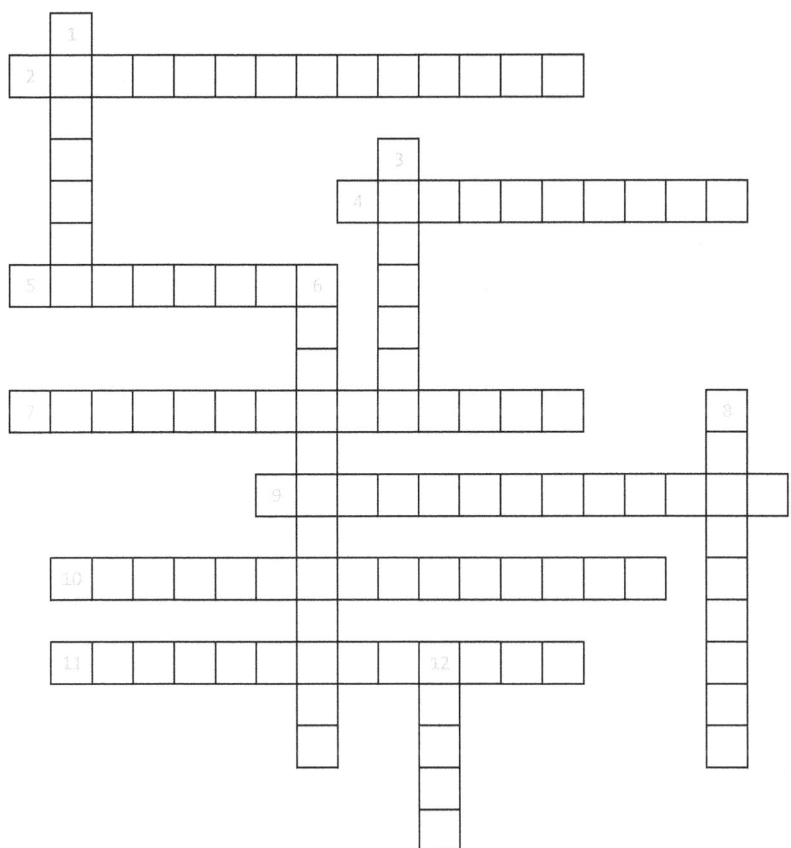

Across

2. Refers to pre-designed forms for recording trial data directly in to an electronic system.
4. An independent personnel or organization, hired for performing a specific duty.
5. The treatment group of a clinical trial.
7. The process of handling the data collected during a clinical trial.
9. Three basic ethical principles: respect for persons, beneficence and justice.
10. Rate and extent of a drug reaching the systemic circulation.
11. The total number of deaths relative to the total population at a specific place in a specific period of time.

Down

1. A part that is a definite fraction of a whole sample for laboratory testing or analysis.
3. A program designed to give supportive care to people in the final phase of a terminal illness either at home, independent facilities or within hospitals.
6. Toxicity studies for 18-24 months in vivo and in vitro are done to assess ____________.
8. The frequency of disease, illness, injury, and disability in a population.
12. The difference between the smallest and largest values of a set of measurements.

Crossword # 129

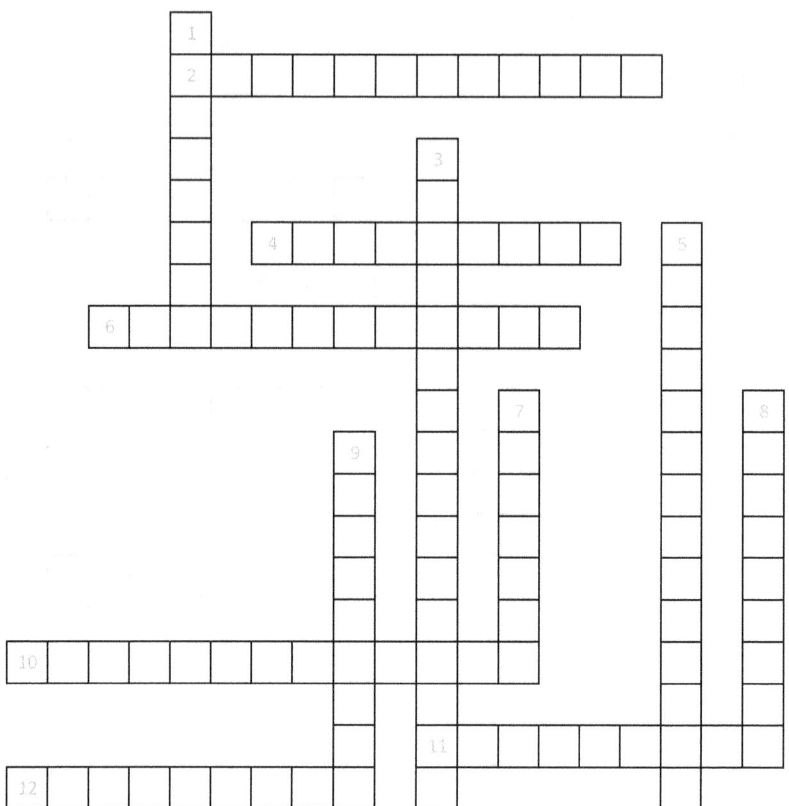

Across

2. Normal value ranges for standardized laboratory tests.
4. The relation of an adverse event (effect) to the study drug/procedure.
6. Storage of data under proper environment and access control, after the completion of a trial.
10. A scale for ranking items where the distance between adjacent points are equal.
11. Refers to a variable that has an influence on another dependent variable.
12. Refer to discovery of a new drug, device, method, process or useful improvement upon any of these.

Down

1. An event or outcome to answer the primary hypothesis of a clinical trial.
3. Planned and systematic actions that are established to ensure that the trial is performed and the data are generated, documented and reported in compliance with GCP and applicable regulatory requirements.
5. The category of drugs that undergo parallel track review by FDA.
7. Refer to Newborn baby.
8. Enteric coating is done to achieve the dissolution of a drug in ____________.
9. The closeness with which results replicate analyses of a sample.

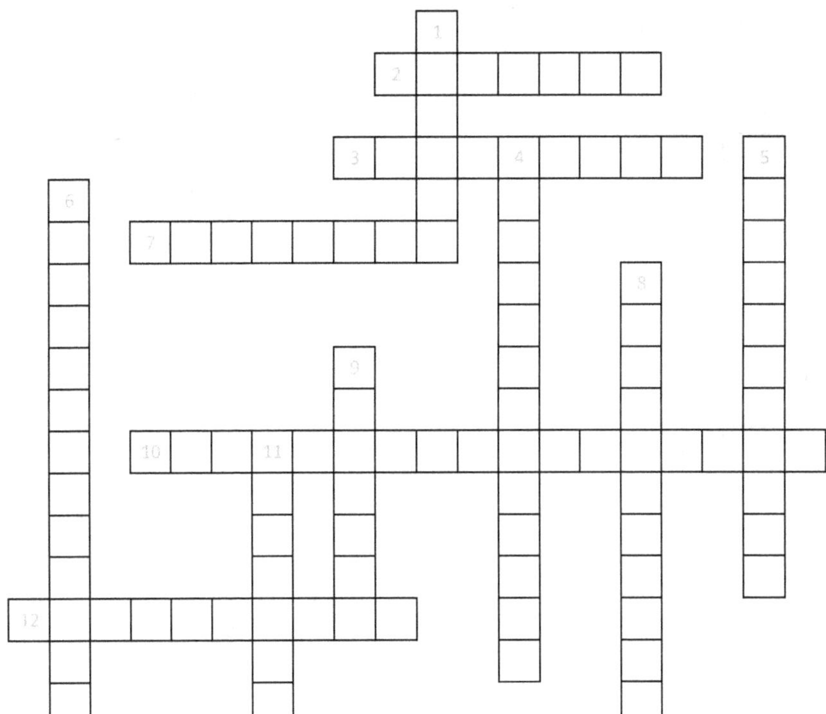

Across

2. The body of a deceased person used for imparting medical education.
3. Refers to any observable characteristic or trait of an organism such as morphology, biochemical or physiological properties.
7. A type of statistical chart that displays the distribution of levels of a categorical variable.
10. A statistical test that provides an analysis of variance by ranks and is the non-parametric equivalent of the F-test for analysis of variance.
12. Cognitive impairment refers to a medical condition in which an individual's capacity for judgment and reasoning is significantly ___________.

Down

1. A document that grants the sole right of an invention to its inventor.
4. A subject matter expert in a peer-group.
5. A medical procedure that doesn't involve skin break.
6. An important factor in the absorption of a drug.
8. The act of transforming document, text or phrases from one language to another.
9. A component or a substance that is analyzed employing an analytical technique.
11. The responsibility of filing NDA (New Drug Application) to the regulatory authorities lies with _________.

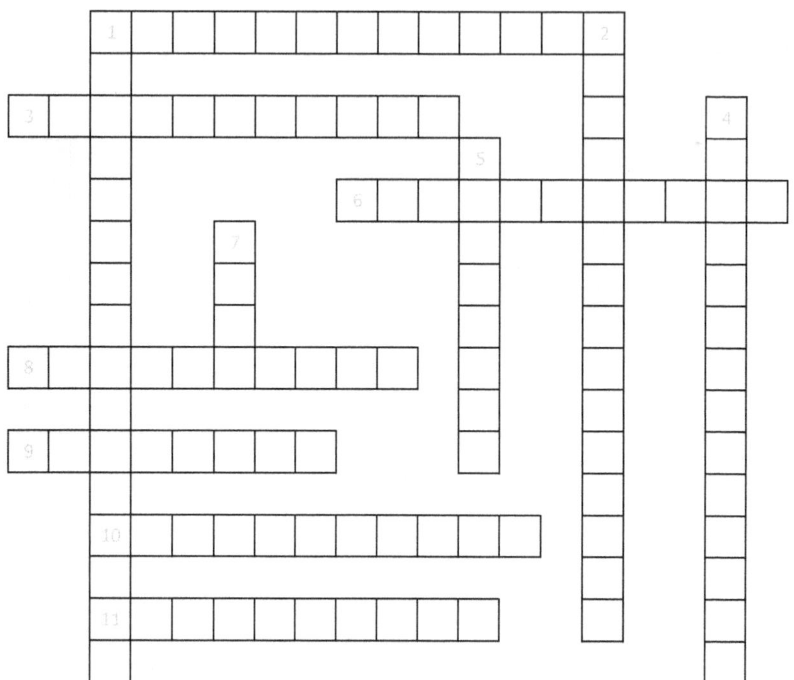

Across

1. Refers to the time period between the initiation and completion of a trial at a site.
3. Clinical ___________ refers to the noting or record of clinical signs and symptoms in a subject.
6. Actual cost associated with an activity.
8. Form 44 represents ___________ to conduct clinical trial in India.
9. Time required to eliminate 50% of the drug from the body.
10. Substances or agents that can interfere with normal embryonic development.
11. Text or numbers generated during the analysis of a clinical trial data.

Down

1. A type of retrospective study comparing persons with a given condition and persons without the condition with respect to antecedent factors.
2. Advertisement for recruitment of study subjects require approval from ________.
4. Documents given to subjects for recording certain observations on the condition of their health, at their home or at trial site.
5. Intensity of an adverse event.
7. A preconceived personal preference or inclination that might influence the assessment of the trial.

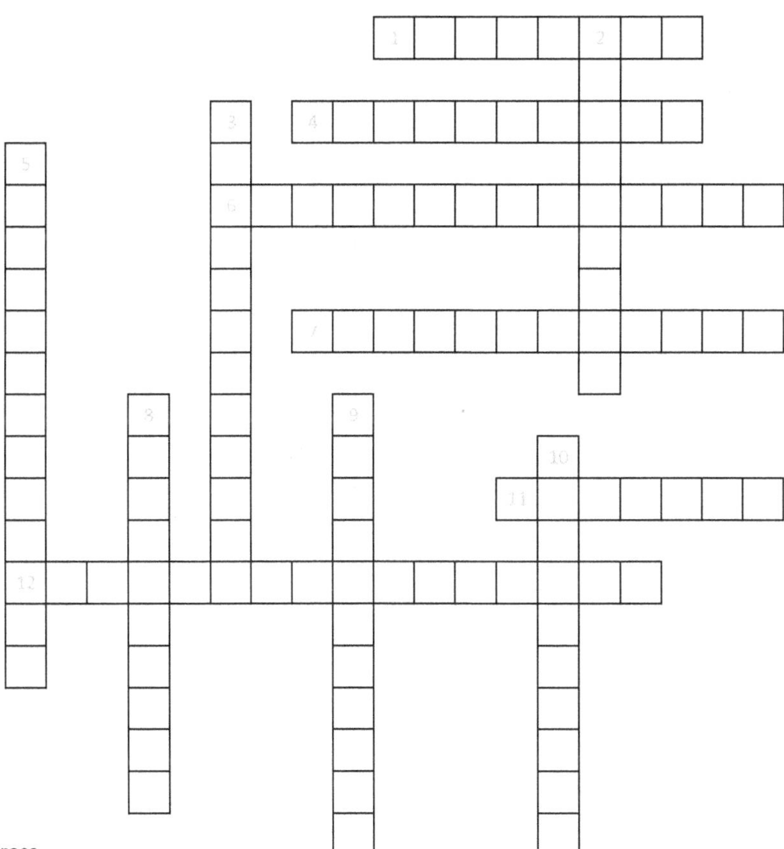

Across

1. Systematic investigation designed to develop new/innovative products, processes or services as well as improvisation of the existing products, processes or services.
4. Characteristic of a drug used to determine crystal morphology and particle size.
6. An authorization to undertake medical practice as per applicable regulations.
7. Supervision of clinical trials by FDA.
11. The principle of moral rightness in action or attitude.
12. A clinical study designed to demonstrate the efficacy of a product.

Down

2. Causative factor for a deviation or event.
3. Payment made to the study subjects for participation in a clinical trial.
5. Refer to the subject that does not respond to the trial drug or therapy.
8. Adherence to study protocol, GCP guidelines and the applicable regulatory requirements.
9. Analytical reports/tables for a given dataset.
10. The documentation of activities that allows reconstruction of the course of events.

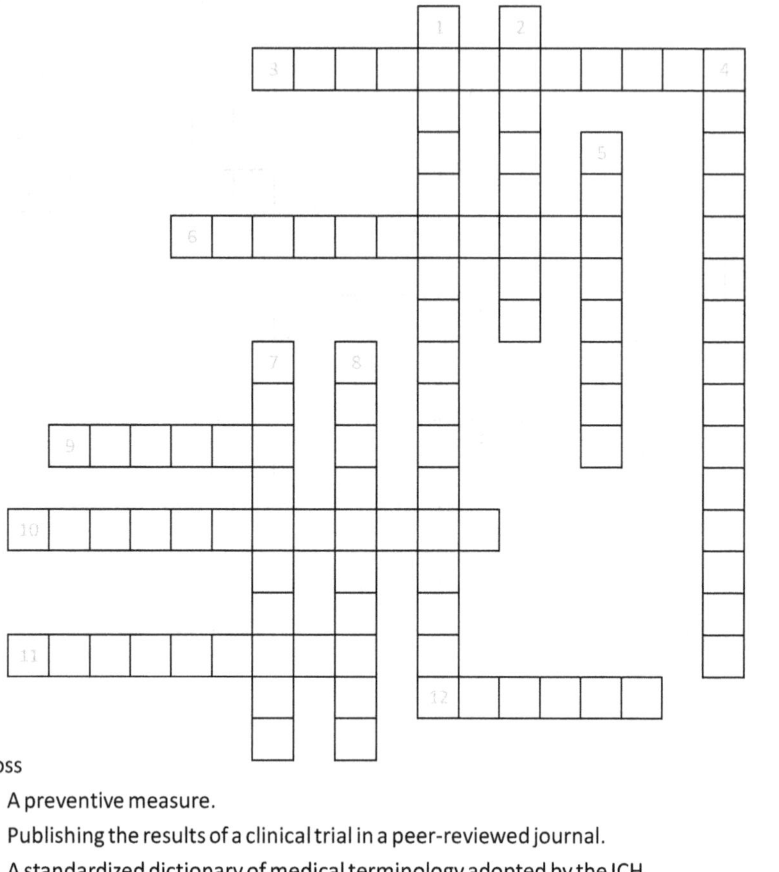

Across

3. A preventive measure.
6. Publishing the results of a clinical trial in a peer-reviewed journal.
9. A standardized dictionary of medical terminology adopted by the ICH.
10. The allocation of specific trial related duties to the individual study team members at the investigator site is the responsibility of ____________.
11. Formal submission of a trial application by a sponsor to the regulatory agency, followed by obtaining no objection for initiating the trial is referred as Clinical Trial ____________.
12. Down coding or down grading is part of ____________ audit.

Down

1. Study of cost-benefit ratio of drugs with other therapies or with similar drugs.
2. Clinical study design in which one or more parties to the trial are kept unaware of the treatment assignment(s).
4. Central value from a series of observation around which all other observations are dispersed.
5. The process of absorption, distribution, metabolism and excretion of a drug or a vaccine in a living organism is referred to as Pharmaco ____________.
7. The act of copying someone's words, ideas, results and presenting them as original content.
8. Refers to the number of people in a given population with a specific condition.

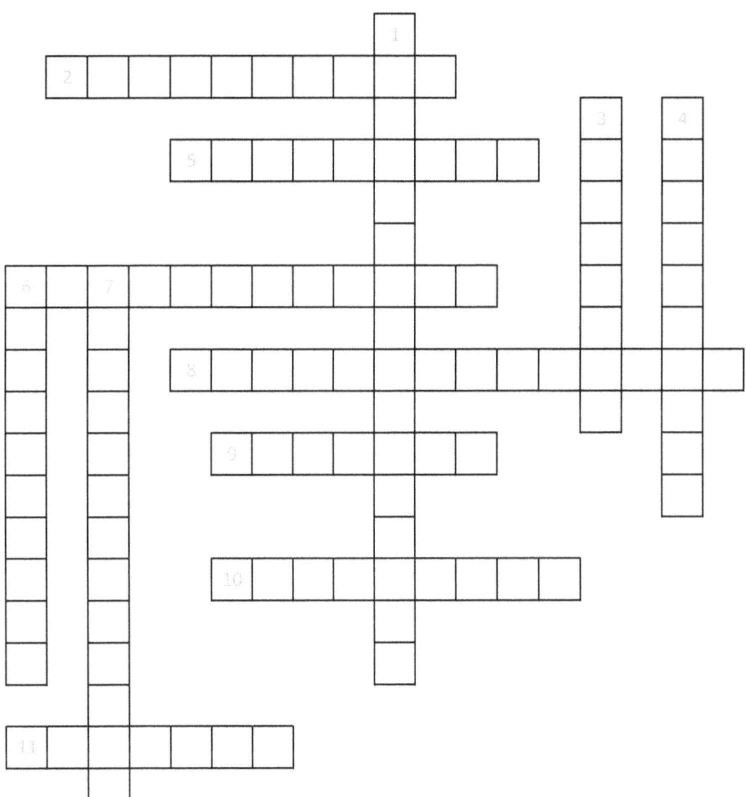

Across

2. Refers to a condition that forms the basis for the initiation of a treatment or of a diagnostic test.
5. A document that contains results of the laboratory tests.
6. An estimate of the total cost implication for carrying out a particular activity.
8. A treatment designed to facilitate the process of recovery from injury, illness or disease to as normal a condition as possible.
9. Means "I shall please" in Latin.
10. A subject who has satisfied the entire protocol requirements and is eligible for the safety and efficacy analysis.
11. Concentration/strength of a drug, at which it is effective.

Down

1. A clinical trial design in which investigational product is compared with an approved drug or placebo.
3. The ability to understand the purpose, procedures, risks, benefits and alternatives to a research study.
4. Codes used by the FDA to classify medical devices according to the potential risks or hazards.
6. United States agreement to cover all Federal sponsored research by a common set of regulations.
7. Data on the stability of a drug product under routine and accelerated stability conditions.

Crossword # 135

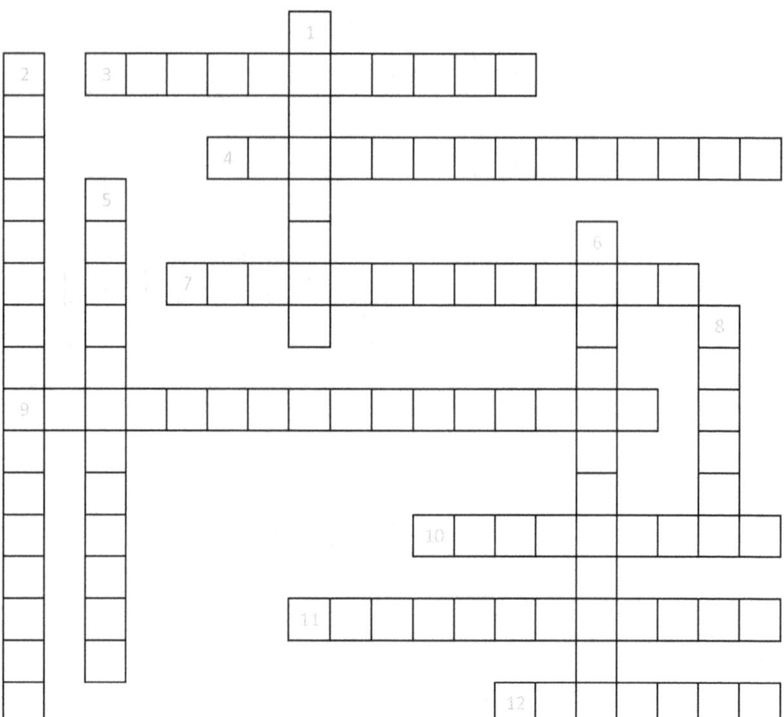

Across

3. Recording and reporting of false data or results.
4. A tool used during the randomization process to ensure an exact balance between the treatment arms with respect to key patient factors that are strongly related to the outcome variable.
7. Primary or secondary outcomes used to judge the effectiveness of a treatment.
9. Process of checking the accuracy of the data that has been entered into a computer database.
10. A new invention.
11. A single legal entity that uses or discloses protected health information only for a part of its business operation.
12. A condition that impairs the normal functioning of an organism or body.

Down

1. Ethical guidelines for biomedical research on human subject.
2. A state in which a person is not able to manage his/her affairs or to make a choice due to a psychiatric or developmental disorder.
5. Constitution of study team at a trial site is the responsibility of ________________.
6. Compounds obtained from High Thoroughput Screening process that demonstrates the ability to interact with the desired target.
8. A computer that acts as a gateway for providing one or more services over a computer network.

Crossword # 136

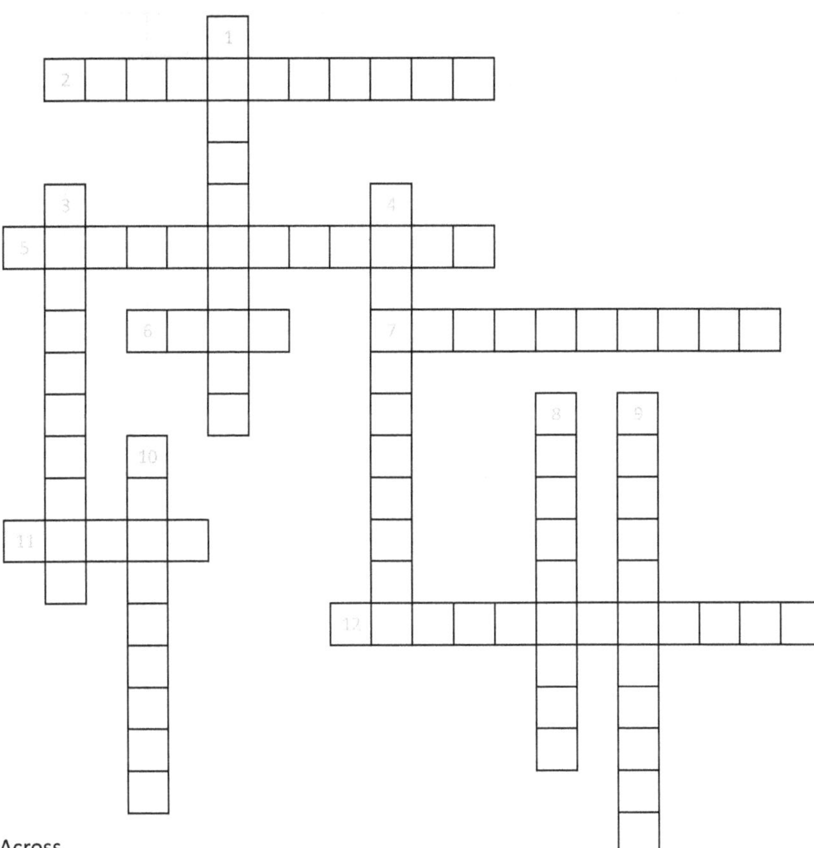

Across

2. A contract to perform a part of or all the obligations of another contract.
5. A set of patient numbers which are grouped together for statistical purposes.
6. An arithmetic value that is obtained by summing up all the observations and dividing by the total number of observations.
7. A list of relevant published literature on a topic along with complete citation.
11. Refers to an individual who has not attained the legal age of consenting to a trial, as per the applicable regulations.
12. Yearly review of the progress of a trial by ethics committee(s) or regulatory agencies.

Down

1. Name of a website/web server.
3. Refers to the documentation of activities that allows reconstruction of the course of events.
4. A measurement of the strength of the relationship between two variables.
8. Time period and storage condition under which a drug is stable.
9. _______ _________Analysis is done to quantify the benefits associated with the use of a particular medication vis-à-vis direct cost implications.
10. ____________ health information refers to any information about health status, provision of health care or payment for health care that can be linked to an individual.

Crossword # 137

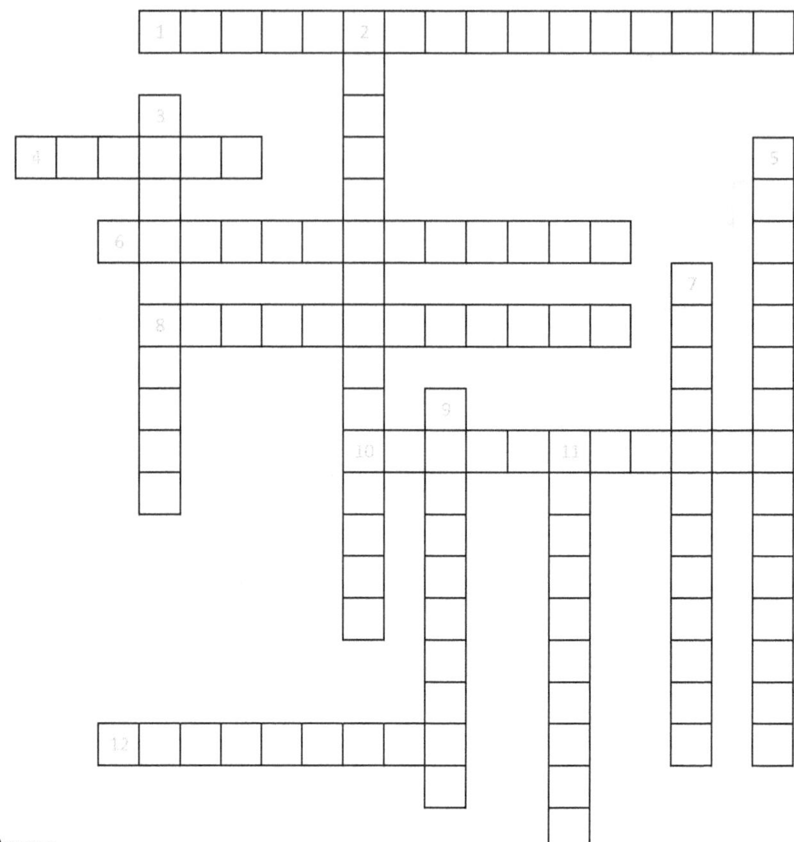

Across

1. A measure of how a subject, feels, functions or survives.
4. __________ requirements must be fulfilled for a valid EC meeting.
6. Report prepared from a serious and unexpected adverse experience.
8. Any untoward medical occurrence in a patient, who has been administered an investigational product and which does not necessarily have a causal relationship with the treatment.
10. Disaster that lead to Kefauver Harris Amendment of 1962.
12. The period of time during which a woman is providing her breast milk to an infant or child.

Down

2. Statistical tests used for drawing conclusions about differences between two or more groups.
3. A systematic and independent examination of trial related activities and documents.
5. Adverse event in which a subject is at immediate risk of dying.
7. A person having knowledge and competence of statistics.
9. An event resulting in death of a subject.
11. A substantial disruption of a person's ability to conduct normal life functions.

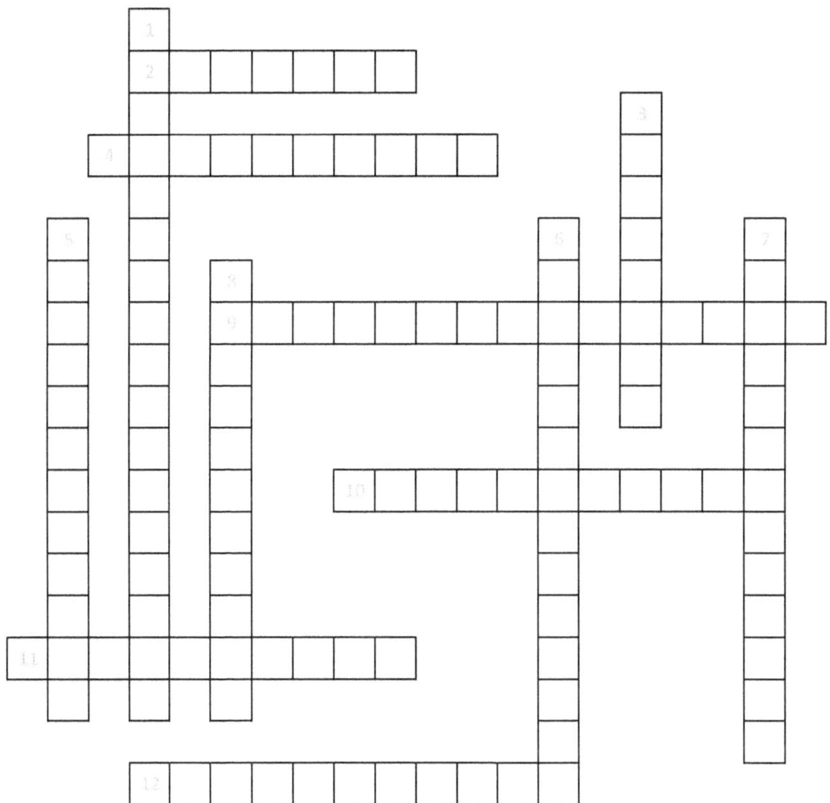

Across

2. Willful oversight in performing a particular activity.
4. All information in original record and certified copies of original records of clinical findings, observations or other activities in a clinical trial.
9. Studies conducted to estimate the rate and extent of drug absorption.
10. A process of estimating the magnitude of some attributes of an object such as its length or weight.
11. Ability to act on one's own behalf, after having understood all the consequences thereon.
12. The notes to explain the deviation/ violation of a particular activity/ process.

Down

1. A novel therapy backed by strong scientific data.
3. Refers to an individual who is legally authorized to consent on behalf of a child for participation in a clinical trial.
5. Primary object of a clinical trial (e.g. drug, vaccine, behavior, device or procedure).
6. Medical management of a patient based on established regimen or guidelines.
7. The accuracy and validity of a given data.
8. Sign, symptom or laboratory results, not characteristic of normal individuals.

Crossword # 139

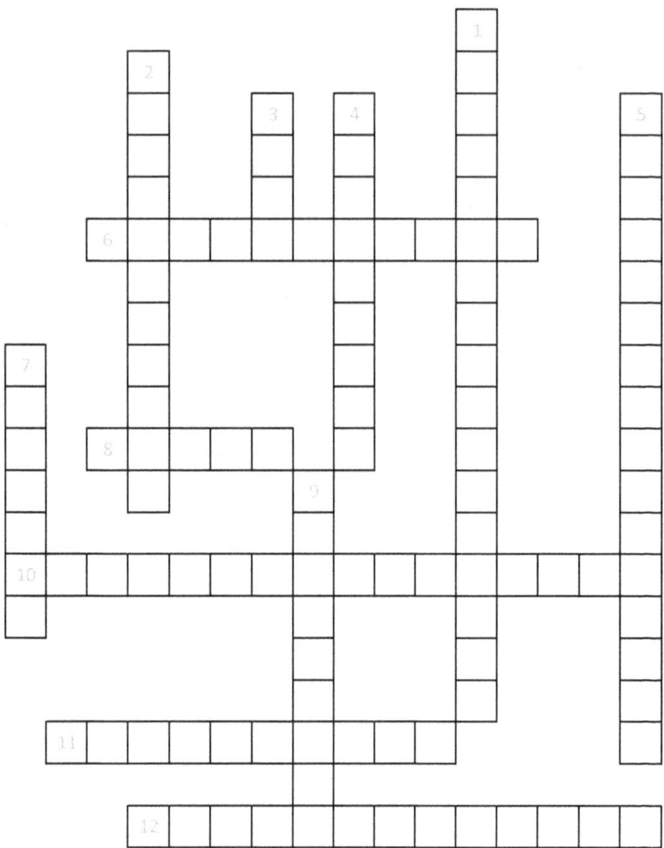

Across

6. A written plan to define the critical project milestones, cost estimate, timelines and deliverables.
8. A systematic and independent examination to determine whether trial related activities were conducted and the data were recoded, analyzed and accurately reported according to protocol.
10. A biological molecule used as a marker to measure the progress of a disease or effects of a treatment.
11. A person with the authority to oversee the work of a person or group.
12. Statistical principle which states that all randomized patients should be included for analysis.

Down

1. Methods for the assessment and prevention of adverse events.
2. A medicinal product with the same active ingredient as that of an innovator drug.
3. The main purpose of Phase-1 studies is to establish a ____________ dosage range.
4. The year in which Declaration of Helsinki came in force is Nineteen________ ______.
5. Trials that are conducted to find better tests or procedures for diagnosing a particular disease or condition.
7. An inactive substance designed to resemble the drug being tested.
9. Refer to intentionally misleading or withholding information.

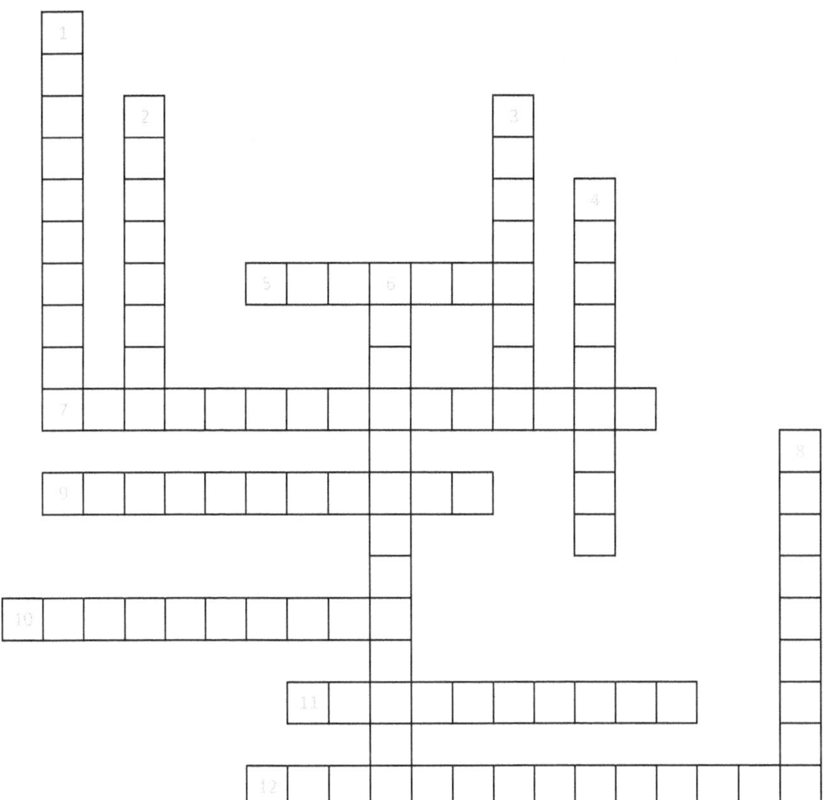

Across

5. Stakeholder responsible for the supervision, coordination and execution of successful data management of a clinical trial.
7. Target Selection is being revolutionized through the application of ________________.
9. A unique identifier assigned to a clinical study for its easy identification.
10. The act of breaking the blinding codes of a clinical trial.
11. An analysis involving a random variable.
12. A file that contains all the essential trial documents at a trial site.

Down

1. Refers to the pharmaceutical delivery system for a drug product.
2. A chemical synthesized or prepared from natural sources that is evaluated for its biological activities in preclinical tests.
3. A formal written agreement which sets forth the working arrangements, between two or more parties.
4. A person who submits a trial application to a regulatory agency.
6. Necessity of informed consent was first described in _____________.
8. Replacing a document with the new one after the same has been revised/ updated.

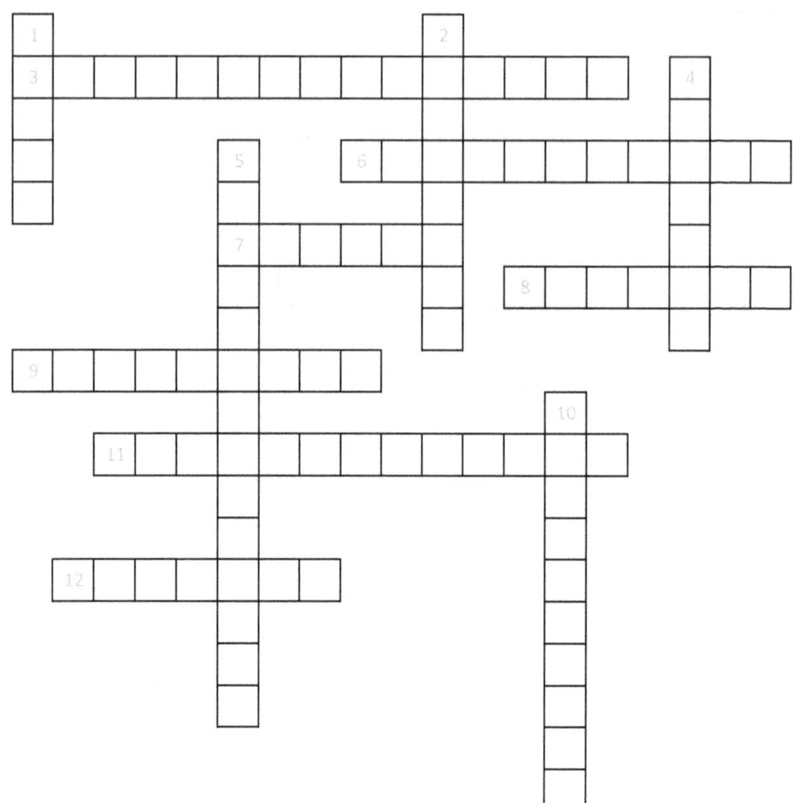

Across

3. A procedure by which certain type of research, involving no more than minimal risk, may be reviewed by the chairperson of the ethics committee or designee, without convening a meeting of the entire EC.
6. Needle placed in the arm with blood thinner to prevent the blood from clotting inside the needle or tubing.
7. A list of topics to be discussed in a meeting.
8. A pattern of black vertical lines containing the coded information to uniquely identify and/or track clinical supplies.
9. __________Trial refers to a clinical trial designed to examine the benefits of a product in real-world environment.
11. Investigation of an approved drug in a new/unapproved indication.
12. Refer to an observation that is numerically distant from rest of the data.

Down

1. A fatal outcome of an adverse event.
2. A pre-designed form/document that includes standard fill-in-the-blank spaces for capturing the standard information.
4. The responsibility of the preparation and submission of Regulatory Dossier lies with __________.
5. The drug products that have the same active ingredient, dosage, form, route of administration, strength or concentration are as called ________equivalents.
10. The act of overseeing the progress of a clinical trial.

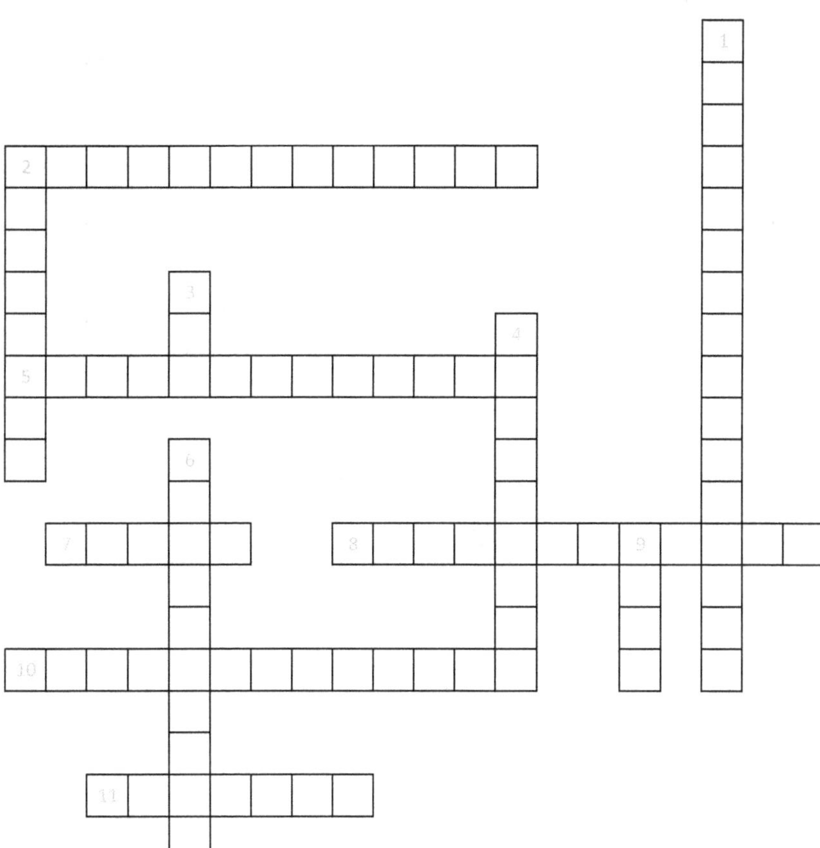

Across

2. Drugs that are approved by a regulatory agency to be marketed in a country.
5. Refer to an article that has a potential to become a successful drug through systematic clinical trial investigations.
7. An act causing physical, social or mental harm or discomfort.
8. Large stocks of clinical trial supplies.
10. Description of the circumstances in which a particular data is required.
11. Deviation from standard operating procedure(s) or the regulatory guidelines is termed as ___________ deviation.

Down

1. The entity responsible for the pharmacological action of a drug substance.
2. A written, formal clarification in an essential trial document.
3. Drugs that are available for purchase without a physician's prescription.
4. The regression of a disease condition.
6. An official review of documents, facility, records and any other resources related to clinical trial by a regulatory authority at the site of the trial.
9. Safety reporting of marketed drugs in a specified period of time (generally on an annual basis).

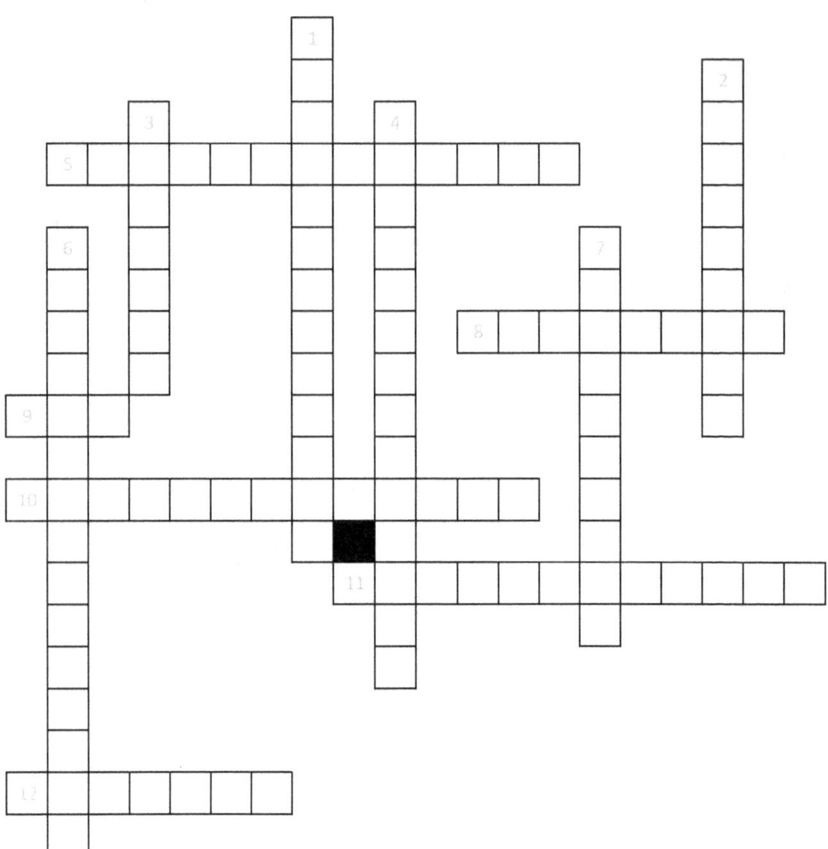

Across

5. A person (18 years of age and above), who is related and has maintained a regular contact with the prospective trial subject.
8. A process to ascertain that management of clinical trial(s) and associated processes, utilize qualified individuals is referred to as __________ Qualification Review.
9. Refers to legislation.
10. Primary or secondary outcome(s) used to judge the effectiveness of a treatment.
11. Potential of a substance to cause cancer.
12. Achievement of a desired outcome in a clinical trial.

Down

1. The code of medical ethics, designed to protect the safety and integrity of study participants and which came as a result of medical experimentation conducted by Nazis during World War II.
2. A query generated during the data entry or review of a clinical trial data.
3. The concentration of a drug at which it is effective.
4. A document that characterizes the data content of a system.
6. Studies that determines the maximum tolerated dose.
7. The process of evaluation of the hardware and software of a system, to ensure accurate and reliable compliance with user requirements.

Across

1. A trial design in which subject is randomly assigned to receive either the standard treatment or the investigational drug.
6. The arm in a clinical trial refers to ___________.
8. The act of signing up participants into a clinical study.
9. The process of assessing the readiness of an investigator site for initiating the enrolment in a clinical trial.
10. A place where drug is prepared and dispensed.
11. A type of study in which both the investigator and subject knows which treatment the subject is receiving.
12. Total surface area of the human body which is widely used for the calculation of drug dosages of cancer medicines.

Down

2. A process by which subject voluntarily confirms his or her willingness to participate in a clinical trial.
3. Technique involving genetic linkage studies and genetic association studies.
4. A person who is independent of a trial, and who witness the adequacy of informed consent process, if the subject and his/her legally acceptable representative are unable to read and write.
5. New Drug Application is filed to obtain marketing _____________.
7. Reporting of ongoing safety, progress reports, and re-approvals to IRB is the responsibility of ___________.

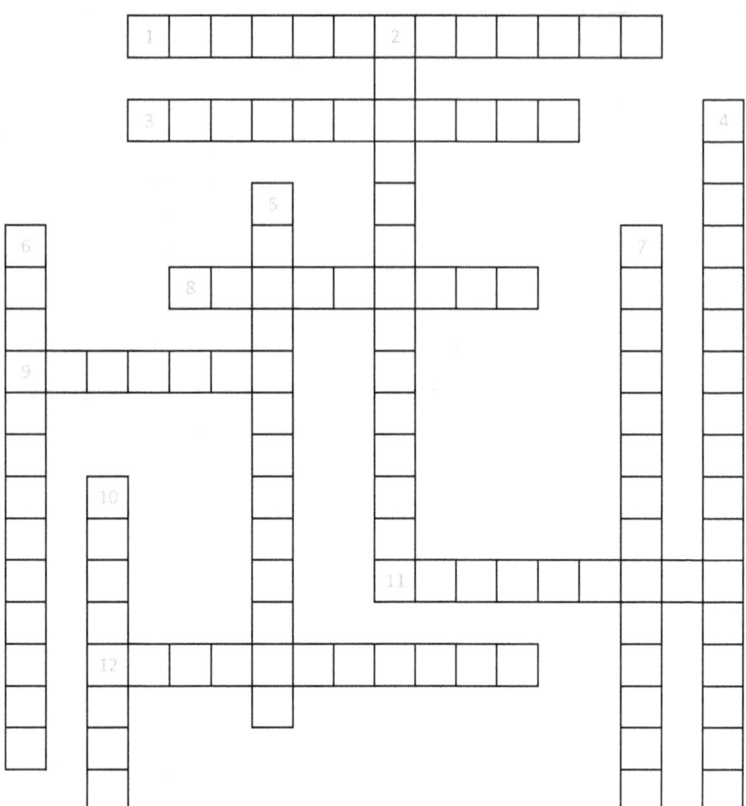

Across

1. Any investigation in human subjects intended to discover or verify the clinical, PK/PD, and adverse reactions of an investigational product.
3. The process of matching one set of data elements, to their closest equivalents in another data set or in a reference dictionary.
8. A trial design in which all the involved parties knows the treatment group to which a subject is assigned.
9. An individual who participates in a clinical trial either as a recipient of the investigational product or as a control.
11. The scientific basis or hypothesis of a clinical trial.
12. Longitudinal studies in which the sample is a cohort.

Down

2. Letter issued by the EC or regulatory agencies granting the approval for conduct of a clinical trial.
4. A document that set forth the payment terms in a clinical trial.
5. A validated data collection form that contains a series of questions to assess an individual's response on a topic/parameter.
6. Recording of false data or results and reporting them.
7. Documents narrating the conversation or discussion between two or more parties for e.g. letters, emails, fax, telephonic logs etc.
10. An adverse effect produced by a drug that is detrimental to the participant's health.

Crossword # 146

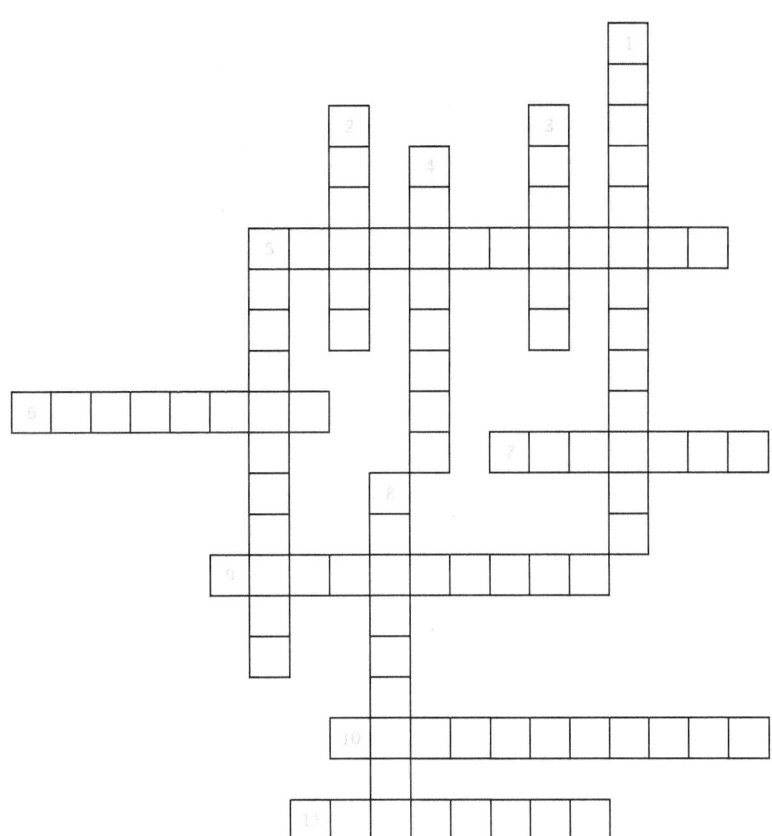

Across

5. Treatment of cancer using chemical agents.
6. A document that describes the objective(s), design, methodology, statistical considerations and organization of a trial.
7. The result of an activity, process, investigation or intervention.
9. Individual identifier based on physical characteristic such as a fingerprint, thumb impression, retina scan etc.
10. ____________ certificate is a document that captures the description and the quantity of a clinical trial material destroyed.
11. Process of converting the data entered in an electronic data entry system to 'read only' format.

Down

1. Assays for the quantitative measurement of a drug, metabolites or chemicals in biological fluids.
2. A process by which a child voluntarily confirms his/her willingness to participate in a clinical trial.
3. Phase II of clinical trials evaluates the efficacy and ________.
4. A written description of a work plan.
5. A type of bias that occurs when the two treatment groups that are being compared, contains different type of patients.
8. Changes made to essential trial documents (such as protocol, ICD, IB etc.) that have an impact on overall conduct of the study.

Crossword # 147

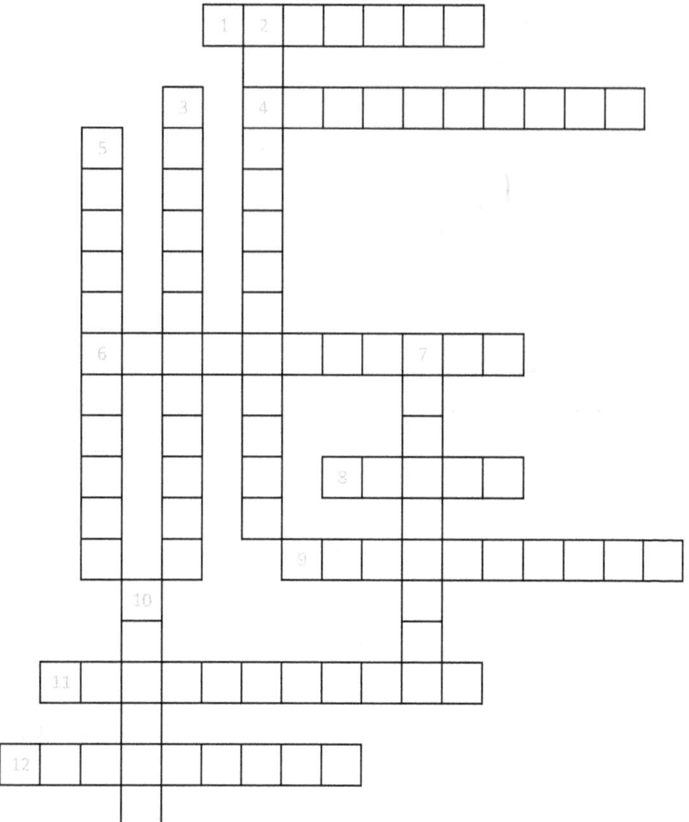

Across

1. A process of submitting competitive proposals to a trial sponsor.
4. An initial study to explore a new hypothesis.
6. The extent of relation between occurrence of an adverse event and administration of a drug/placebo.
8. ANDA does not require incorporation of animal and ________ data to establish safety and efficacy.
9. The process of collecting, recording and summarizing data that is collected from experiments, records and survey.
11. The act of enrolling subjects according to the inclusion/exclusion criteria.
12. Individuals who participates in a Phase-1 clinical trial or a BA/BE studies.

Down

2. The care provided to patients when they are admitted to a hospital or health care centre.
3. A well controlled, randomized study to evaluate the safety and efficacy of a new drug in patients with relevant disease condition.
5. A quality control process of standardizing the equipment, machines, apparatus to be used in scientific testing.
7. Refers to the waivers that are provided under special circumstances with appropriate documentation of authorization.
10. Process of making a copy of important data, onto a different storage medium.

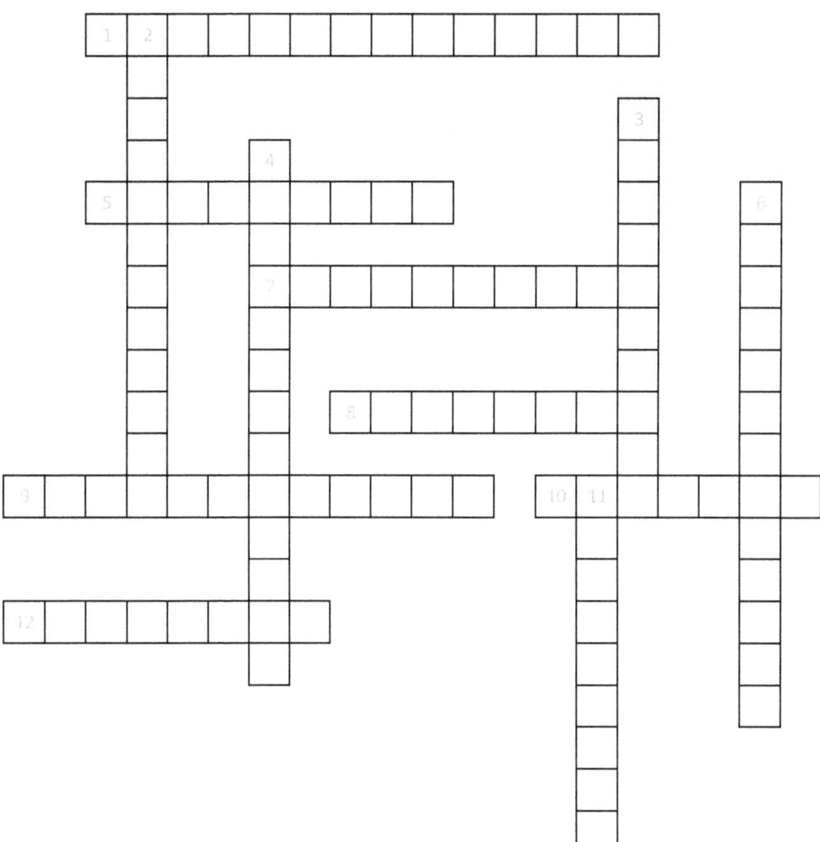

Across

1. Collection of information about each subject during the course of a trial.
5. A law which excludes the users from using original works of authorship, fixed in any tangible medium of expression.
7. A set of rules for streamlining processes according to a set routine.
8. Unacceptable subject recruitment involving undue inducements, duress or indirect pressure to participate in a clinical trial.
9. The science of drug and their clinical use is called clinical ______________.
10. Blinding is also known as ________.
12. Refer to time scale.

Down

2. An official communication from regulatory bodies to trial sponsor/investigator/EC, documenting its decision.
3. An objective or goal to be achieved in a stipulated time-frame.
4. A drug discovery approach that involves finding a drug or group of drugs which works on the selected targets.
6. A validated data collection form that contains a series of questions to assess an individual's response on a topic/parameter.
11. A person who submits a trial application to a regulatory agency.

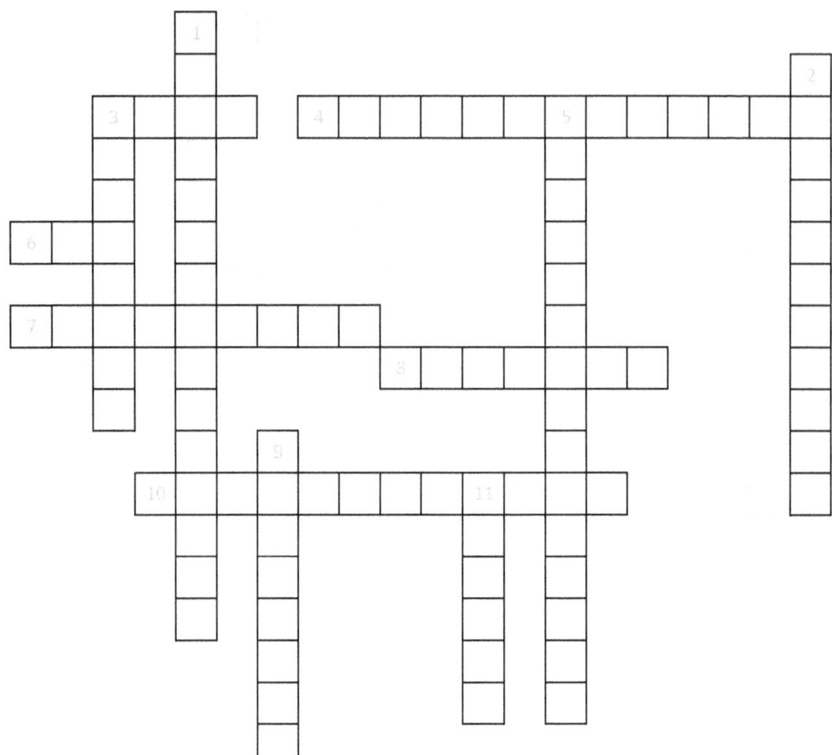

Across

3. The main purpose of Phase-1 studies is to establish a ______ dosage range.
4. The process of assigning trial subjects to treatment group using an element of chance.
6. Application filed to regulatory agencies for initiating phase I trial.
7. A name, word, symbol or phrase used to identify a particular product.
8. Pilot clinical trials to evaluate safety in selected patient populations.
10. Primary object of a clinical trial (e.g. drug, vaccine, behavior, device or procedure).

Down

1. Adverse event in which a subject is at immediate risk of dying.
2. Any public or private entity or medical or dental facility where clinical trials are conducted.
3. The treatment group of a clinical trial.
5. A process by which subject voluntarily confirms his or her willingness to participate in a clinical trial.
9. Intensity of an adverse event.
11. Convenient and commonest drug dosage form.

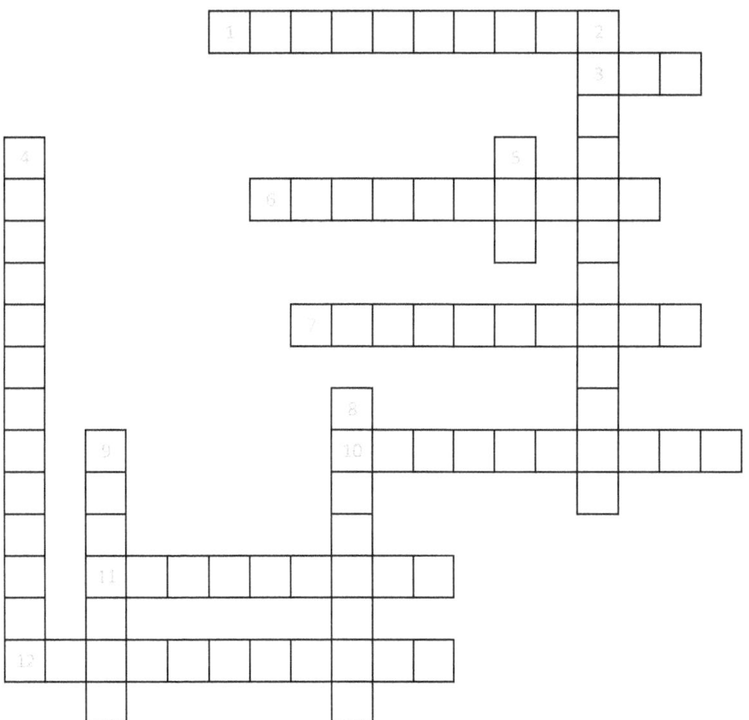

Across

1. An analysis involving a random variable.
3. Drugs that are available for purchase without a physician's prescription.
6. Adherence to study protocol, GCP guidelines and the applicable regulatory requirements.
7. The research in an institution that is supported by external funding is known as ____________ ___________ Research.
10. A government order with the force of the law.
11. De-identified information of a trial participant that in no way can disclose his/her identity.
12. Time period for which the patent of a drug is valid.

Down

2. Data on important co-factors associated with a disease state.
4. Primary or secondary outcomes used to judge the effectiveness of a treatment.
5. A classification of regulatory inspection outcome that does not require any action or response.
8. Storage of data/records at the end of a trial for a stipulated timeframe.
9. The body of a deceased person used for imparting medical education.

2

Jumbled Words

In this section you will find **160** Jumbled Words pertaining to clinical research. You have to identify the correct word and mention it in the relevant empty boxes. The solution should fill all the empty boxes for a particular jumbled word and may contain widely used abbreviation of the original term also.

Scoring: Excellent (able to solve ≥144 jumbled words); Very Good (≥128 to <144 jumbled words); Good (≥112 to <128 jumbled words); Satisfactory (≥80 to <112 jumbled words); Unsatisfactory (<80 jumbled words).

1. SCBTAART

A	B	S	T	R	A	C	T

2. TCUCNIOLBAIYAT

3. EARIDCCIATNOT

4. AEDDNMDU

5. DSAEVRE

6. AAGNED

7. MMNANEDTE

8. PLORVAPA

9. AVRAHCIL

10. STNAES

11. TUIDA

12. UASYTPO

13. LESABIEN

14. SBAI

15. IALABITLOIYBIAV

16. BIAIAVABELOL

17. BOCFNSAOMITRII

18. IOCRBITSME

19. POSNYSIS

20. TIBIATOSSTSCI

21. LOCOETIGHBNOY

22. NLDIB

23. LBGDNIIN

24. OTABCAILRNI

25. IERCNGIOACCN

26. CTSAAYULI

27. IICCALNL

28. GDNOIC

29. OHCRTO

30. ORMROAATPC

31. AELCPOINMC

32. TIONACCOTMN

33. TIATIEDYNONCIFL

34. OCTSNNE

35. RIIAAIONNOTTCNCD

36. CONORTL

37. CIATOORRLEN

38. SOVSCRROE

39. EADASATB

40. ODAEIITVN

41. CEIVDE

42. ISSDIGNAO

43. ESOCDYIRV

44. SSEIADE

45. ENAUMDOOINTCT

46. DSOE

47. RTPODOU

48. URDG

49. FYEICFAC

50. RIIALECPM

51. TIPENNDO

52. ODPYLEIIMGOE

53. EISTCH

54. UXSEIOLCN

55. EELENAXIMRPT

56. FAD

57. TFLMIOANURO

58. ENGILEIUSD

59. HATSILOP

60. HSOEYTSHPI

61. SNIUOICLN

62. TNNDIOIAIC

63. TCSENIPOIN

64. TICERATNONI

65. IENTTNOEIVRN

66. NEASIVVI

67. ETSGAIIVTONR

68. BLALE

69. YRORLABAOT

70. LTCOISGIS

71. CURAMNSITP

72. EKMDAS

73. ENEDIIMC

74. MLASMBOEIT

75. NRMOGNIITO

76. AMORYTILT

77. AEUTMGNCI

78. ERUMBNREG

79. OTERIBAVSALNO

80. LOTEURI

81. PENTTA

82. NIPATTE

83. TIPHSRCMAA

84. INASMAODCPHCMRAY

85. EOCCINMPAOSMROHCA

86. AMPARKCTHCIISNEO

87. CHMPALOYAOGR

88. LNACAVIEIPGHRMAOC

89. RPHAAMCY

90. SPIHACNIY

91. BEOPALC

92. PMGNRSOTKAIET

93. PTOYECN

94. LRPCILENIAC

95. CIRPTNRPOSEI

96. ELVCRAEPEN

97. PECORJT

98. CIPROHATLCPY

99. ARSLPPOO

100. PVPSETRICOE

101. OLOPCRTO

102. YAITUQL

103. QIRSEUINATEON

104. MNRAOD

105. NRODMITANOAZI

106. AOAINTRLE

107. CTEINMEURTR

108. SRRCEEEENF

109. MEGNRIE

110. ITENUROGLA

111. GYOULTRERA

112. RRTPEO

113. RAESEHRC

114. EVSECRTETOPIR

115. TSFAEY

116. CERINGSNE

117. SOERCU

118. ICSTISNAIATT

119. UTJBCSE

120. SEEPSURDE

121. ETPELAMT

122. OTTREEIAGCN

123. PAYRTEH

124. XIICTYTO

125. RNSOILANTTA

126. TTANMRETE

127. ILRAT

128. IBNUNIGNLD

129. VLITDIAONA

130. SEIRVON

131. RLTOUNAYV

132. NRUOLETEV

133. LEURLEBAVN

134. OLBMTEN

135. BAIS

136. YTAIAUSCL

137. RRAIOODTCNO

138. ROTPONIEAS

139. YTACSALT

140. OCRTNTAC

141. DEOGAS

142. RARTEAUMLX

143. NBCAOATRIFI

144. GRTNA

145. EMAIFDNNIIINOTC

146. TSCOCIMNUD

147. KSRI

148. OMPSTMY

149. YRSVEU

150. TIWSENS

151. LCINEUETRTM

152. HESPA

153. OSRNSEEP

154. TESAG

155. LROONTC

156. TDTASAE

157. NIPDAERCCSY

158. RLELON

159. EROYLPXATRO

160. LTPAIAMIR

3

Word Search

In this section you will find **31** exercises containing 10 words each pertaining to a particular clinical trial element/activity/process. You have to identify the 10 words in each exercise and encircle them. You could find these words either upwards, downwards or diagonally.

Please note that the solutions could be,

i. A single word (e.g. Site) or more than one word (e.g. Site Initiation),
ii. A widely used abbreviation of the original term

Scoring: Excellent (able to solve ≥27 exercises); Very Good (≥24 to <27 exercises); Good (≥21 to <24 exercises); Satisfactory (≥15 to <21 exercises); Unsatisfactory (<15 exercises).

1. Clinical Project Milestones (i)

J	N	B	K	P	E	W	R	X	Z	K	J	T	K	C	S	Z	Q	F	E
K	U	Q	P	R	Z	J	F	M	S	T	E	D	U	H	K	W	Z	L	Z
V	Q	M	H	O	U	B	A	C	K	K	R	K	A	P	P	A	A	R	V
N	W	V	N	J	U	V	X	O	Z	Y	N	A	U	U	N	V	Y	G	W
I	K	K	P	E	J	U	J	K	A	B	P	T	D	E	O	R	M	R	O
P	F	I	K	C	J	M	D	U	Q	K	E	R	C	R	Z	N	N	U	U
P	A	Q	A	T	D	V	P	T	X	S	E	T	P	O	V	G	D	L	O
R	W	I	D	P	C	H	K	X	E	L	O	P	R	W	T	A	H	D	O
O	S	M	H	L	T	S	B	S	A	C	A	I	A	A	Y	X	K	H	S
C	D	G	K	A	M	C	A	D	N	Y	L	W	T	T	I	P	Q	G	P
U	M	V	O	N	X	B	T	K	R	A	D	T	I	H	I	N	K	Y	F
R	N	B	E	M	A	C	G	O	R	I	V	L	Z	D	I	M	I	I	P
E	J	C	F	T	P	L	T	A	T	T	I	M	T	V	F	W	D	N	V
M	Y	N	A	T	Z	A	I	V	A	B	L	R	Q	Z	S	C	J	P	G
E	Z	D	H	R	L	V	Y	X	I	Q	Z	Z	R	G	F	I	S	D	H
N	R	Y	U	U	O	F	C	S	W	G	Z	W	R	S	O	U	V	B	R
T	D	S	G	J	I	R	A	I	M	A	F	Z	R	O	D	H	P	O	D
W	M	E	F	C	T	E	F	W	E	C	A	P	P	R	O	V	A	L	S
K	R	V	X	G	F	S	I	T	E	S	E	L	E	C	T	I	O	N	B
T	I	E	J	N	E	S	T	W	N	R	J	U	Y	X	A	Y	S	B	R

2. Clinical Project Milestones (ii)

L I Q I X J S W L F U P Z T B R L V I Y

M N X F E A A V E F Y W B T T T Q H N Z

D Z Q P R L S A X H E B Y V N R Z M T C

A M B N O K F Z R F N Z P E O P F V E F

T T H T T I A M N C E L M D K D U F R Q

A K F H B G R F G N H E I K K A F Y I D

L Q A C V S M L B W G I Z S W P U F M Z

O R U K C M F W F A T C V D F U N I A G

C B O H N I F Y N E H N O A V B D U N T

K Z K K Y P G A P B D L L X L L R F A T

E O X A D J M L Q B Z V Z Z T I F T L T

H D N F W A J X U N C U C B E C Z V Y Y

S D S I T E C L O S E O U T N A C G S L

K P C A Q H T P E V M R F A E T T R I C

N Z D X Y A O M B B W W H L S I W M S Z

O W R H C L E X U U X I N Z C O H U G L

L D H U W T R I A L C L O S E N U A C N

W M T V L P N K H D O X L I R A R I B E

3. Ethics Committee

H	U	N	N	A	U	S	O	A	P	P	R	O	V	A	L	N	R	H	I
G	B	O	B	Z	S	O	A	Q	G	V	P	Q	A	S	Z	I	Z	N	H
X	B	D	C	O	K	F	D	W	T	K	Y	W	N	T	P	X	E	F	D
E	W	X	U	W	L	Q	J	H	A	V	E	W	W	Z	B	A	N	V	G
Q	I	N	I	T	I	A	L	R	E	V	I	E	W	K	F	K	L	Y	D
I	Q	F	Q	G	Y	T	L	V	H	M	N	J	U	F	H	T	A	Q	M
J	F	S	X	J	X	M	L	P	I	S	Z	A	H	E	C	U	Z	V	C
U	F	A	V	O	R	A	B	L	E	O	P	I	N	I	O	N	U	K	D
T	F	D	I	S	A	P	P	R	O	V	A	L	R	T	T	O	E	T	Y
X	H	L	W	Z	X	M	F	N	W	V	H	R	D	B	F	Q	I	U	Z
I	W	W	M	F	Y	P	D	Q	Q	P	M	P	O	S	M	S	V	E	I
C	K	X	E	D	V	T	T	B	J	V	D	T	R	C	E	I	F	I	C
A	Z	C	V	X	E	X	P	E	D	I	T	E	D	R	E	V	I	E	W
R	B	V	R	X	Z	N	C	X	Z	U	B	V	I	M	N	F	W	G	G
Q	U	O	R	U	M	Y	E	D	X	M	C	H	S	K	G	U	Z	D	X
N	Y	I	K	X	U	A	F	G	E	Y	U	P	M	B	X	K	E	B	H
D	C	P	S	S	O	D	Y	M	A	X	Z	Y	C	Q	E	J	H	R	B
A	R	O	K	W	N	X	A	J	R	L	O	X	W	C	Y	P	V	Z	V

4. Investigational Product

E	Y	G	S	S	Z	K	N	U	M	G	K	M	D	S	Q	J	B	R	K
C	O	A	Y	J	S	Y	F	N	O	I	G	G	Z	G	D	P	G	G	U
D	X	N	H	E	H	S	J	M	T	H	W	I	N	M	Y	H	A	N	J
E	A	L	B	N	Z	N	H	N	E	Y	O	I	Z	P	O	X	H	N	G
S	G	R	O	S	R	I	Q	I	M	C	S	Y	K	H	R	A	Q	A	R
T	M	J	M	U	Q	T	K	M	P	N	G	A	D	X	G	A	B	C	E
R	I	V	T	X	Y	D	K	X	E	M	I	U	J	E	V	E	Q	C	C
U	A	E	Z	B	M	S	H	P	R	F	E	S	K	R	C	Y	U	O	E
C	R	Q	S	L	N	H	S	P	A	O	X	N	X	Q	S	O	K	U	I
T	B	X	T	O	S	I	J	N	T	B	R	Q	T	Z	X	C	E	N	P
I	U	S	O	X	D	B	U	W	U	T	D	C	I	X	H	R	X	T	T
O	I	D	R	A	Y	Z	J	J	T	H	S	Q	H	W	G	B	P	A	Q
N	Y	V	A	E	B	F	V	D	R	R	Y	E	R	N	O	T	U	B	S
M	V	U	G	R	N	K	D	U	E	M	R	U	O	M	P	D	V	I	U
G	V	U	E	Z	E	V	W	S	L	L	X	J	N	V	J	A	Y	L	Z
L	D	J	Z	W	D	I	F	R	O	U	W	B	W	I	X	Z	D	I	Z
U	X	D	X	Z	U	Z	V	H	G	F	R	G	Q	M	Z	H	L	T	Q
K	G	A	R	W	A	C	C	E	S	S	C	O	N	T	R	O	L	Y	I

5. Clinical Trial Monitoring

M	I	M	H	H	B	S	A	E	R	E	V	I	E	W	M	P	I	T	D
O	Y	P	F	W	J	R	X	J	Y	S	Z	H	F	Q	L	U	P	J	X
N	O	R	R	X	N	D	Z	Y	J	C	R	F	R	E	V	I	E	W	I
I	N	D	L	O	M	O	F	A	W	X	A	G	H	M	Y	N	B	F	A
T	T	G	S	A	T	U	C	R	H	G	I	X	S	V	D	A	H	E	D
O	F	X	C	K	U	O	T	Y	U	L	O	W	C	G	W	J	A	R	E
R	N	Z	N	V	I	P	C	S	I	N	A	D	W	X	K	S	S	X	V
I	A	S	D	W	I	H	G	O	M	A	F	R	U	D	Z	V	A	C	I
N	V	S	A	C	R	F	C	O	L	L	E	C	T	I	O	N	Y	Q	A
G	H	S	T	P	O	V	N	A	Y	C	C	H	D	F	Q	E	H	H	T
R	Y	V	F	I	T	R	S	B	K	P	O	I	T	I	O	J	G	B	I
E	D	I	T	B	T	N	T	S	I	B	T	M	L	W	D	R	R	O	O
P	S	L	A	Q	P	D	C	J	V	X	Z	H	P	N	A	U	G	V	N
O	G	S	D	C	Q	V	Z	A	P	N	Q	V	T	L	O	C	Q	F	S
R	E	G	U	L	A	T	O	R	Y	C	O	M	P	L	I	A	N	C	E
T	C	O	R	I	A	E	X	Z	G	C	E	F	N	D	D	A	C	H	Z
M	I	P	A	C	C	O	U	N	T	A	B	I	L	I	T	Y	N	R	E
F	Z	Y	F	K	O	H	N	L	M	C	V	K	V	W	F	E	Z	C	L
E	O	J	Y	H	J	Y	I	C	D	R	E	V	I	E	W	Z	W	L	E

6. ICH-GCP Required Elements for ICD (i)

R	Y	I	W	Y	A	L	C	O	M	P	E	N	S	A	T	I	O	N	S
S	A	Q	L	X	E	C	L	B	G	U	J	A	C	F	C	A	P	T	L
T	Z	L	E	O	N	B	G	J	V	X	T	Y	B	S	S	G	I	T	S
U	E	F	T	K	P	A	W	B	P	K	B	M	T	L	R	F	G	R	F
D	U	O	W	E	G	R	P	U	R	P	O	S	E	Q	E	G	I	I	C
Y	M	R	G	S	R	D	O	M	L	V	U	Q	Q	N	X	F	B	A	Z
P	F	E	D	Y	R	N	O	R	S	N	S	P	E	O	A	K	Y	L	J
R	Z	S	Y	D	Q	L	A	E	A	S	X	B	Y	A	P	L	L	T	D
O	O	E	P	F	E	E	Y	T	S	T	D	T	L	U	K	K	A	R	U
C	G	E	Y	P	C	D	R	D	I	E	E	H	J	S	F	Y	F	E	X
E	F	A	O	U	Q	C	C	Q	T	V	X	D	R	J	R	X	X	A	K
D	W	B	D	X	X	Z	D	C	A	K	E	C	P	A	Z	W	Z	T	L
U	A	L	L	E	X	P	E	N	S	E	S	C	T	A	I	T	V	M	C
R	H	E	B	M	J	P	I	Y	Q	F	B	N	O	D	Y	W	U	E	I
E	H	R	K	F	X	H	K	A	P	M	U	F	N	U	L	M	A	N	K
O	P	I	N	E	K	U	T	Q	Y	L	W	O	U	N	R	D	E	T	Z
V	B	S	C	N	P	L	V	A	O	M	T	S	D	C	O	S	L	N	V
Q	I	K	X	T	M	W	C	V	K	Q	L	W	B	O	Z	M	E	C	T
Q	S	S	Q	G	A	D	K	G	E	C	J	W	B	D	P	F	G	G	H

7. ICH-GCP Required Elements for ICD (ii)

S	E	G	N	N	T	T	R	B	Y	W	V	K	Z	B	P	X	A	T	L
F	M	T	R	E	S	E	A	R	C	H	S	T	U	D	Y	S	C	X	Q
E	E	D	A	O	N	V	I	F	C	P	P	U	W	H	T	E	X	R	A
R	R	J	R	R	B	A	S	K	Z	Y	R	B	C	C	P	A	F	A	N
I	G	C	E	V	Z	S	L	T	B	R	J	A	E	S	K	L	T	N	V
G	E	R	O	Z	I	K	L	G	O	U	H	J	A	N	K	V	O	D	Q
H	N	U	W	N	S	Z	B	E	B	V	B	L	R	X	I	J	V	O	R
T	C	V	N	J	F	M	V	G	V	U	A	P	S	D	H	T	I	M	M
T	Y	B	Y	R	Y	I	P	B	S	T	P	U	Q	X	W	R	R	A	M
O	C	T	Q	A	K	E	D	F	N	Q	D	Q	Z	S	D	Z	J	L	J
R	O	I	I	K	U	B	O	E	L	K	K	Y	R	A	J	F	Q	L	Z
E	N	J	V	S	T	R	M	K	N	E	D	F	T	T	H	R	I	O	I
F	T	J	O	C	E	I	C	Z	M	T	S	U	I	C	J	J	T	C	I
U	A	P	W	B	R	J	N	K	B	G	I	T	R	D	Q	J	K	A	M
S	C	A	M	E	A	T	Z	B	X	D	R	A	I	A	O	D	B	T	D
E	T	U	P	X	S	R	C	A	E	E	C	T	L	P	T	F	N	I	N
Y	N	X	A	R	J	J	R	S	S	T	K	D	W	I	C	I	U	O	O
V	E	I	J	T	E	R	M	I	N	A	T	I	O	N	T	S	O	N	Y
R	E	S	P	O	N	S	I	B	I	L	I	T	I	E	S	Y	X	N	G

8. Clinical Trial Stakeholders

A	D	R	D	K	Y	U	H	S	S	Y	E	A	I	T	Q	K	I	I	S
K	R	R	E	L	Z	D	T	L	P	E	J	D	S	P	R	J	N	Y	M
H	U	A	X	G	C	B	M	I	H	V	Y	C	P	R	Y	G	V	F	O
N	F	Y	V	J	U	S	U	K	G	M	N	E	O	I	P	C	E	F	S
T	T	Y	R	F	P	L	T	K	Q	M	I	T	N	W	S	N	S	K	U
V	E	P	E	T	O	W	A	U	H	Z	I	C	S	M	I	P	T	L	S
N	E	D	C	K	X	V	G	T	D	N	N	P	O	T	Q	E	I	J	G
P	J	D	M	R	O	D	G	F	O	Y	N	Z	R	A	R	N	G	L	K
H	K	Q	F	U	B	J	F	M	C	R	S	X	W	S	J	L	A	M	X
Z	T	P	H	V	O	Y	Y	C	A	M	Y	U	P	P	I	Y	T	L	D
Q	S	O	E	R	N	D	N	W	I	U	J	A	B	G	I	I	O	Z	O
K	G	A	O	V	U	H	I	C	W	F	I	D	G	J	Z	T	R	Q	K
K	D	V	D	T	R	X	R	B	Q	P	I	Y	D	E	E	X	N	G	B
K	C	U	S	T	F	O	Z	W	M	K	E	M	L	H	N	C	F	P	G
K	W	R	O	H	T	X	M	F	A	E	H	X	M	M	R	C	T	Q	B
A	S	U	B	I	N	V	E	S	T	I	G	A	T	O	R	T	Y	S	J
I	T	N	D	G	F	K	H	Y	M	N	Y	I	B	H	J	E	I	I	T
S	C	U	Q	N	I	C	R	O	D	H	R	T	B	S	F	J	Y	R	Y
J	A	K	T	F	C	M	D	G	W	A	O	F	I	K	P	R	O	B	Z

9. Sponsor's Responsibilities (i)

Y	A	O	M	D	X	I	P	M	A	N	A	G	E	M	E	N	T	M	N
W	B	W	Y	Y	D	Z	N	O	V	T	V	I	F	T	X	I	I	O	P
J	K	B	N	B	Q	A	H	D	O	Z	P	D	N	B	T	P	I	X	O
R	S	Z	S	X	I	X	T	R	K	B	T	E	M	U	K	T	S	L	C
B	R	S	A	I	U	K	W	A	O	F	M	E	S	O	C	W	W	D	R
Q	I	L	R	R	R	I	H	D	M	P	U	S	P	E	W	Q	N	Q	A
L	B	J	R	X	F	B	T	T	O	A	A	K	L	O	V	A	M	X	G
H	X	E	X	O	U	S	E	L	Q	F	N	E	Z	V	N	O	Y	T	R
M	J	X	G	U	H	H	E	H	H	I	S	A	R	J	N	T	N	A	E
M	K	B	W	V	Q	V	C	L	B	E	I	P	G	S	M	A	E	L	E
I	L	S	D	D	E	N	S	F	T	M	J	W	H	E	A	E	D	D	M
L	B	A	S	D	M	H	V	I	D	C	D	J	J	K	M	I	L	N	E
K	H	R	D	E	X	F	S	S	V	G	F	P	A	D	G	E	D	R	N
B	G	C	L	K	A	T	R	I	A	L	P	L	A	N	N	I	N	G	T
O	I	S	T	I	F	O	X	K	W	E	U	U	E	V	E	T	Z	T	S
P	R	O	T	O	C	O	L	D	E	V	E	L	O	P	M	E	N	T	F
B	R	Q	H	K	P	U	B	L	I	C	A	T	I	O	N	D	M	W	T
T	M	T	R	I	A	L	M	A	N	A	G	E	M	E	N	T	T	O	O
Z	R	E	G	U	L	A	T	O	R	Y	A	P	P	R	O	V	A	L	Q

10. Sponsor's Responsibilities (ii)

D	C	R	F	D	E	V	E	L	O	P	M	E	N	T	U	S	M	G	Q
N	C	V	A	I	L	T	A	B	S	H	Q	E	U	G	H	S	N	C	J
P	O	J	S	Y	L	G	O	Y	A	J	F	L	G	L	T	I	M	Y	W
V	M	Q	G	I	X	Q	L	D	F	N	Z	X	O	F	T	P	I	E	K
P	G	Z	V	M	R	B	S	I	E	U	T	E	J	I	A	P	Q	V	L
B	A	X	N	V	C	Y	H	L	T	H	I	K	D	M	O	F	Z	K	N
X	P	Y	I	L	N	K	I	S	Y	Z	R	U	M	K	I	X	Y	V	R
G	L	C	M	L	B	E	D	E	R	R	A	E	S	I	A	W	Q	X	P
W	T	C	T	E	L	O	S	H	E	R	R	Z	E	B	H	W	H	X	F
B	R	J	Y	O	N	C	S	R	P	R	E	P	A	R	A	T	I	O	N
P	B	C	F	Z	V	T	R	E	O	H	L	N	C	M	U	T	C	Y	R
J	R	B	T	M	H	Q	S	P	R	X	H	W	N	O	F	H	R	S	C
I	N	V	E	S	T	I	G	A	T	O	R	T	R	A	I	N	I	N	G
J	E	A	H	P	Y	V	K	N	I	Z	P	M	K	X	B	H	G	S	R
Q	J	N	T	F	U	W	M	O	N	I	T	O	R	I	N	G	B	F	R
O	A	R	E	M	P	D	Y	E	G	D	A	S	D	N	M	E	H	E	R
G	P	E	R	I	O	D	I	C	R	E	P	O	R	T	I	N	G	J	S
P	O	I	B	D	E	V	E	L	O	P	M	E	N	T	Q	K	I	S	L
T	G	C	P	C	O	M	P	L	I	A	N	C	E	J	N	L	W	Q	U

11. Investigator's Responsibilities (i)

Q	D	T	K	R	A	D	S	H	M	J	M	W	X	F	Y	Z	E	J	R
I	A	G	O	U	I	P	A	B	P	T	W	D	V	I	E	C	S	Y	G
C	T	C	S	H	D	C	F	R	X	M	M	X	D	Y	N	H	O	P	C
D	A	P	E	Y	R	B	E	E	B	G	F	J	B	E	K	T	U	E	Z
A	C	C	P	O	T	M	T	C	Z	M	R	I	D	S	J	G	R	R	O
D	O	O	N	I	V	Q	Y	O	B	O	B	N	S	M	A	J	C	I	I
M	L	M	A	K	E	I	R	R	Q	N	O	O	P	Y	O	G	E	O	P
I	L	P	K	U	Z	Z	E	D	Q	P	D	H	S	Z	D	P	D	D	M
N	E	L	N	M	B	K	P	R	S	S	P	S	Y	W	Y	I	O	I	A
I	C	I	F	M	C	E	O	E	S	B	L	G	K	N	O	T	C	C	N
S	T	A	F	M	R	G	R	T	C	N	U	B	Z	D	I	Q	U	R	A
T	I	N	C	V	U	R	T	E	U	M	A	K	U	N	I	N	M	E	G
R	O	C	U	O	O	A	I	N	X	V	T	K	N	K	L	G	E	P	E
A	N	E	Z	C	Q	N	N	T	Y	E	K	R	I	L	J	O	N	O	M
T	Z	U	B	G	M	Y	G	I	B	K	C	P	S	B	H	T	T	R	E
I	B	R	N	V	N	N	S	O	U	T	O	E	M	J	P	S	A	T	N
O	I	M	P	N	J	Q	L	N	T	W	V	Z	H	C	R	M	T	I	T
N	V	N	N	M	E	D	I	C	A	L	C	A	R	E	I	O	I	N	L
E	U	X	T	Y	N	X	V	X	B	Z	G	H	G	S	Y	Y	O	G	A
S	M	K	C	W	I	Q	E	J	L	P	I	I	M	O	X	F	N	S	I

12. Investigator's Responsibilities (ii)

K	V	Q	E	E	Y	G	U	W	Z	J	T	I	Z	J	A	Q	T	E	A
S	P	A	T	I	E	N	T	C	O	U	N	S	E	L	I	N	G	S	C
R	W	G	V	V	T	E	W	N	L	G	W	B	I	V	V	J	E	Q	C
V	J	R	D	K	R	W	I	O	L	Q	G	Z	F	F	Z	I	I	W	E
T	M	E	O	B	T	Q	V	L	S	I	G	Q	I	N	T	A	E	V	S
D	O	E	M	F	S	Z	R	U	S	E	U	L	Q	U	L	Y	Q	D	S
A	X	M	M	B	S	L	Q	I	P	H	H	A	D	Q	I	E	P	C	C
D	A	E	X	E	X	K	E	N	O	Q	C	F	L	N	J	Z	F	F	O
W	F	N	A	K	C	D	M	A	U	U	O	A	D	D	E	G	G	R	N
D	Q	T	B	D	N	H	C	L	U	N	V	P	Z	G	I	M	J	E	T
Z	J	S	Q	Z	D	X	R	B	O	I	R	N	I	V	J	B	X	S	R
U	C	L	Z	D	S	X	F	I	H	L	J	X	D	R	S	C	T	O	O
H	H	R	R	E	B	O	T	C	S	J	L	M	K	I	O	P	N	L	L
T	E	S	Z	E	O	A	R	H	V	U	T	H	V	R	M	S	Y	U	F
N	K	E	P	E	C	A	P	X	H	Y	S	I	Z	A	K	T	U	T	E
A	M	W	R	O	C	R	F	C	O	M	P	L	E	T	I	O	N	I	D
I	N	Q	L	Z	A	D	R	M	A	N	A	G	E	M	E	N	T	O	S
C	M	L	V	R	H	A	K	X	L	O	B	Z	V	I	B	L	Z	N	O
T	A	P	R	O	T	O	C	O	L	C	O	M	P	L	I	A	N	C	E
C	O	N	F	I	D	E	N	T	I	A	L	I	T	Y	J	M	Z	M	F

13. IRB Responsibilities

D R G W A B X N X H F D H Y E B J W D B

A P E F A R N I Z T R C W M F C F R O R

G R I V M C O M P O S I T I O N I I N L

Y V G M I X V V D Z C V R C W R S T X R

Z E C S N E L A V V Q V U Q T L C T W E

T X P L U C W J N M J A B Z Q T Q E G C

R P C M T J V O F W O M L O O O I N J O

I E O B E O I Y F R T L C B N V R P I R

A D M Q S J W B L D V G U I E S H R N D

L I P G O K S O E F O C I R K W J O I R

A T L W F Y O L K Z D C G G P Z F C T E

P E I B M S N M N X R N U F U M O E I T

P D A N E S L U Q C I A Q M R R O D A E

R R N L E I U V R U K L Y R E E K U L N

O E C U T U E O N B X D F P P N U R R T

V V E M I V J I L M E Z Y L M W T E E I

A I X V N T T A Y Q D U P W H V F S V O

L E B N G N Y K Y V X O O D Q V E D I N

B W R R O T O N K E M Q K Y Z A E L E A

H A I C H B M K A C T Q W G Z H D V W H

14. Documents Required for Initial IRB Review

M	M	A	S	G	C	J	T	Z	K	K	E	B	N	Q	J	O	D	B	T
K	E	D	Y	A	V	L	Z	Q	G	S	I	Z	L	V	L	C	F	S	E
D	S	V	V	K	F	K	O	F	D	X	E	R	G	Q	I	T	Q	O	I
Z	U	E	R	N	U	E	F	T	B	B	A	Y	L	A	N	I	G	O	S
S	W	R	K	V	V	L	T	F	X	T	M	N	K	E	O	P	H	B	X
M	Q	T	K	P	S	K	H	Y	S	I	O	G	M	B	J	N	Q	H	S
I	Z	I	B	Y	U	M	B	V	I	H	Y	E	S	S	N	V	P	N	F
N	D	S	B	X	B	C	V	H	P	N	E	O	R	H	H	J	O	B	X
V	O	E	H	U	J	V	F	U	S	R	F	Z	W	B	F	I	S	A	I
E	O	M	C	M	E	V	W	H	G	V	E	O	V	L	T	V	E	N	E
S	J	E	O	I	C	G	O	A	I	H	O	I	R	A	I	F	O	E	K
T	A	N	F	U	T	Z	L	I	L	O	Y	Q	L	M	N	Y	F	N	B
I	M	T	Q	U	D	A	N	R	B	F	U	S	O	V	A	R	H	E	U
G	E	S	D	P	I	G	X	B	V	T	N	S	K	W	D	T	P	Z	K
A	M	A	X	R	A	T	C	J	H	A	W	Y	H	B	X	R	I	B	A
T	Q	P	T	B	R	R	K	I	R	A	M	C	J	X	J	U	A	O	Z
O	V	G	K	O	I	U	U	T	P	K	E	Y	W	S	H	T	K	D	N
R	T	G	S	Y	E	Y	D	E	N	Z	I	B	R	B	N	U	J	E	A
C	H	A	G	H	S	C	R	B	P	R	O	T	O	C	O	L	M	T	O
V	V	H	Z	R	I	I	N	S	U	R	A	N	C	E	G	U	T	F	L

15. HIPAA (i)

Z	G	Y	V	D	C	A	X	W	N	I	Y	J	O	P	U	L	D	M	Z
U	F	D	D	Z	B	F	C	M	Q	R	C	L	Q	X	H	U	H	M	Z
N	O	W	S	A	V	L	A	X	V	E	J	P	D	F	J	Y	Q	A	G
O	E	C	B	M	C	Q	F	U	F	O	G	H	G	V	S	Q	T	F	M
Y	O	G	O	W	I	R	I	C	T	E	V	E	N	B	S	A	P	J	N
T	G	H	P	V	O	N	G	W	O	H	D	U	E	K	D	T	R	S	P
H	J	A	E	A	E	I	I	U	T	F	O	A	Q	C	T	F	N	R	R
A	J	P	I	A	V	R	S	M	X	G	O	R	I	F	X	J	B	H	E
M	G	L	R	N	L	X	E	J	U	V	D	H	I	R	R	J	Y	K	Z
G	P	X	D	I	N	T	S	D	I	M	P	P	V	Z	I	P	P	J	Z
Q	D	S	B	B	V	S	H	L	E	A	S	N	T	Y	A	P	N	Y	J
Q	F	W	U	H	E	A	L	P	R	N	N	T	G	N	O	T	X	X	G
T	E	Z	Y	R	U	L	C	G	L	X	T	X	A	P	H	I	I	B	U
V	I	I	D	F	P	F	O	Y	L	A	X	I	G	N	B	V	J	O	U
C	H	D	V	J	H	M	Q	T	R	T	N	O	T	T	D	M	C	J	N
F	A	P	B	E	E	L	U	Z	I	U	C	S	K	I	O	A	V	K	W
E	L	H	E	D	K	I	T	S	M	S	L	K	C	W	E	L	R	H	Z
L	G	D	B	T	J	N	A	M	E	S	T	E	S	N	D	S	E	D	E
P	E	Z	I	T	Y	V	B	A	F	Q	N	O	M	W	R	O	H	S	S
J	N	C	L	E	A	R	I	N	G	H	O	U	S	E	S	R	L	K	Y

16. HIPAA (ii)

F	K	C	F	Y	P	C	I	Q	K	B	J	I	U	H	R	Q	D	H	I
L	U	V	I	Z	V	Z	K	G	T	A	O	H	O	E	O	Y	M	E	T
O	L	L	R	F	X	V	C	B	J	M	Z	A	B	H	R	B	X	A	A
X	Z	E	L	Q	R	B	P	P	Z	V	B	M	W	A	Y	I	O	L	V
W	D	K	R	F	Z	X	F	Z	S	T	U	Y	S	S	T	O	I	T	X
R	Q	K	V	N	A	I	U	F	H	N	H	S	L	K	W	M	X	H	H
R	Q	S	K	J	Q	C	O	M	E	H	E	W	D	W	O	E	L	C	F
P	Y	C	X	Y	X	K	E	N	A	C	G	X	P	X	H	T	G	A	G
O	B	V	F	E	S	Z	O	P	E	H	Z	U	D	W	L	R	D	R	I
R	P	V	C	Z	C	H	M	N	H	P	G	S	U	F	Y	I	T	E	H
T	C	I	K	V	P	B	M	H	B	O	R	C	D	P	J	C	X	P	W
A	C	H	Q	E	U	U	U	H	I	I	T	W	H	P	E	D	V	R	G
B	J	E	L	I	M	O	J	J	A	E	P	O	K	F	A	A	K	O	V
I	X	E	V	I	X	D	T	K	Y	C	G	K	G	L	W	T	P	V	Y
L	T	P	N	H	Q	Y	O	F	S	T	Y	W	C	R	P	A	C	I	U
I	E	I	I	T	P	E	N	A	L	T	I	E	S	Y	A	L	M	D	Z
T	M	V	Y	I	D	T	Z	A	Q	H	Z	T	O	B	H	P	Y	E	G
Y	C	E	L	E	M	E	N	T	S	O	F	D	A	T	E	S	H	R	U
M	F	M	A	F	R	Y	F	E	M	A	I	L	A	D	D	R	E	S	S
S	N	M	P	X	V	D	R	F	A	X	N	U	M	B	E	R	J	L	T

17. Approaches to Drug Discovery

L	E	M	Q	B	J	U	I	Y	Q	I	Q	V	Q	B	Y	M	Z	B	N
I	M	J	U	D	G	O	E	C	V	E	C	B	G	S	M	S	X	O	P
D	F	E	D	P	H	X	X	L	N	X	B	G	M	M	E	H	I	R	R
M	T	Y	D	M	M	T	R	O	O	F	B	K	U	T	O	T	X	O	E
K	C	V	G	N	E	W	D	R	U	G	M	G	A	T	A	P	U	S	C
O	L	N	L	L	U	J	Z	A	P	X	U	D	X	Z	D	D	G	T	L
Z	I	N	J	R	Y	O	R	Q	W	N	I	O	I	G	R	R	B	X	I
H	N	C	R	F	G	B	J	G	X	D	Q	M	J	N	U	U	Z	V	N
I	I	L	K	V	Y	C	C	H	N	U	I	S	C	K	G	G	M	R	I
T	C	Q	D	V	T	C	E	A	M	T	R	R	S	X	S	C	T	P	C
C	A	D	C	A	L	Z	C	K	P	G	M	S	T	R	E	A	I	Y	A
O	L	Q	U	I	H	D	Z	O	M	M	A	V	X	N	L	N	Y	Y	L
M	T	U	L	M	A	A	D	U	G	O	Y	T	O	H	E	D	A	J	T
P	E	A	E	E	L	A	O	G	W	U	L	D	U	X	C	I	G	G	E
O	S	P	L	P	E	V	U	L	Y	V	G	V	I	N	T	D	C	M	S
U	T	E	V	L	N	O	Y	D	S	A	O	X	E	Z	I	A	Q	K	T
N	I	M	H	T	S	O	K	H	M	O	F	K	P	E	O	T	O	R	I
D	N	K	J	V	V	Y	P	Y	K	G	H	E	V	D	N	E	R	M	N
S	G	U	B	T	A	R	G	E	T	S	E	L	E	C	T	I	O	N	G
M	H	W	F	B	W	C	W	X	T	A	I	Y	K	G	O	T	G	R	Y

18. Clinical Trial Support Service Providers for the Sponsor

S A J N O Y T A T D R U G D E P O T C C
E V E N T M A N A G E R S I X E O T E E
L T G Q T K V K J N O K S M K M Y C N N
I D H A R Z P S R E W J X T S C P O T T
G Y X I O S A F U J P L L I N E T U R R
W B J M R Z M U J D O Y Z E O C W R A A
S D W B P D C U L O L N G V I J X I L L
W C E H E V P W U A Y A N R G U T E L D
X P Z M V Z X A U F N N C R O J R R A I
C W C A S C Y X R O T J V C Q A E A B A
W O A R A W K D I T Y Z B I K V B G Q G
L Z N P Q T C T U X Y T S U U Y H E N N
T L P S Y K A J C U I A B W A L U N Y O
D V G L U L B O F R U L R D Y V H C K S
T M T R S L V S W J O R Q C J O F Y K T
V R A N Y X T W B E I O Q U H G I D K I
I W A F Z W K A V Q N R V K P I G N B C
J R A L V P X V N B U E J B J R V Z R S
T B G P Y E G H Y T L K K E F I F A L V
O M R T F B A F W N S O I A Z Q X Y L T

19. Data Management

X	S	H	Y	S	V	H	G	M	K	Q	H	A	H	X	T	O	D	Z	D
M	Z	P	A	J	P	N	R	A	Z	L	G	V	F	B	D	C	O	L	V
Q	U	E	R	Y	R	E	S	O	L	U	T	I	O	N	Y	A	U	P	T
M	Q	U	K	S	R	J	D	S	Q	U	J	L	N	Y	G	C	B	B	U
W	F	J	F	R	B	Q	A	K	U	U	T	G	Q	B	K	F	L	E	D
D	A	X	G	Q	T	A	T	V	C	M	O	A	O	F	E	T	E	O	J
A	U	L	Z	E	R	Z	A	P	E	D	C	Y	M	P	C	G	D	H	W
M	R	I	Z	D	A	M	B	R	J	R	F	N	J	X	L	Q	A	V	A
A	H	C	E	V	D	M	A	W	A	Q	N	W	H	X	I	C	T	D	Y
T	Q	M	Z	L	H	Q	S	H	C	J	O	C	W	W	N	T	A	O	X
K	I	H	G	N	C	Z	E	N	Y	O	E	R	Q	V	I	P	E	H	O
J	Q	A	U	H	C	F	D	A	T	A	L	O	C	K	C	U	N	T	V
J	R	P	W	L	Q	Q	E	G	U	M	O	E	P	V	A	V	T	H	T
L	H	J	I	A	C	U	S	G	W	A	E	W	E	Q	L	Y	R	T	O
Z	H	W	R	T	R	F	I	R	K	I	T	L	B	M	C	D	Y	A	R
L	P	W	K	Q	R	K	G	S	T	T	H	T	X	Y	O	W	V	O	R
G	G	C	B	S	L	C	N	F	C	F	G	T	D	D	D	M	S	P	B
D	V	D	C	E	U	W	C	F	T	R	L	G	I	K	I	F	T	R	X
P	Z	Z	X	R	O	D	W	W	W	F	F	Y	L	D	N	P	K	O	Y
M	A	Y	V	K	X	P	P	O	X	T	R	G	Q	W	G	M	H	D	C

20. Seious Adverse Events

W Q I L D Y W R Z Q P D I Q Z Q M T O X

X U R K S E T X X T K Y K K S G O X D K

Q B K P C U C A N I L S P N P C F Q Y D

F L C X G E B H O U H E S F E P L I Y X

M O I B P R A J A T T V Y G M C V L M G

T A V F D Y X J A L D G N D O O A Z W H

I L X E E L E E Z K L E G A I M L G S O

E D V F W T D P E L L E H I O P R N V S

Q I U C A K H X S L Q Q N N E L E M Z P

W S N Z R D S R A A I V A G H I A E Y I

I A Y Y S S S H E K E L P N E A S H I T

I B Y K S R C R B A A F Q X R N T W R A

K I W T N E G S V T T B O S V C K T R L

W L M T R G K J I O X N M R C E I X K I

N I H D U X H N S U O O I U M Q A D H Z

H T H G C T E W Q N I M V N C O A R E A

O Y M Z P G Q D J C H E G A G M D I G T

I R W C N D J A N A A U N V F Z R K I I

W J J O X X B T P I M T R H L S Y B L O

N Q C K Z V A W W X W S Q G V L M W M N

21. Regulatory Authorities

H A L W Q D C D G A I B F W Z T D H Z Z
G F W H K J X A H P C U W W M J B S I O
P B L I W R H R O L B H S R Z J P Z D O
P L Z R S T D C G I Y T P F L I C B D I
J X E M V K P T X S O T B D D K R N N N
W H U T G I U Z Z V C Q P L J A O Q K R
B A W C M L I S D T D U Z O Y I F K A F
G F Q W I H C N Y Y A S P K S P R R Z A
D M E C N W O E O O N Z B S N S I J D U
V M T U S I I N O F D O I P Z T L N X N
I D S G P K Z Q O G A M U N Z D N Y N D
E L F Z E E G H K G R F A K P M H R A Q
D P D A C P K R S E U P G M E A B V J W
T E C S T O P Q P E N T C D X E Z C Z R
Y E O D I V J L X E O C A A J V Q W O N
F S S Y O E A J B M Z R Z Y B Y K B M M
R G N A N I E X C E J J G T U C I Q F M
L X D A R O F V T A N N S P T C N N R E
M Q G T R S S A O X N K G J D C D Y A O
G T L W F M H P O I T J K V S X Q N X Z

22. Pharmacovigilance (i)

B	E	I	R	H	H	L	Q	P	E	J	W	Y	Q	Y	I	S	B	Y	J
S	F	N	S	V	E	M	P	R	O	E	R	W	H	G	P	E	A	O	R
K	U	E	W	A	D	Z	C	I	P	L	Q	Q	L	D	R	R	C	C	V
U	H	S	W	L	E	K	M	G	A	U	C	J	L	X	D	I	W	D	C
B	G	M	A	K	A	I	B	F	X	K	R	J	F	O	D	O	X	S	H
O	T	C	D	R	T	C	S	B	D	I	P	M	G	Y	U	U	V	F	G
D	Y	N	X	W	W	A	W	H	W	M	X	Q	F	C	C	S	X	N	U
A	B	U	N	E	X	P	E	C	T	E	D	W	T	G	Y	N	X	K	N
G	H	W	H	R	C	M	V	I	C	B	B	V	K	L	U	E	Z	M	L
O	O	F	A	V	H	D	A	T	V	Y	S	W	F	G	K	S	V	X	I
X	X	L	T	A	D	V	E	R	S	E	E	V	E	N	T	S	I	E	K
V	C	T	V	S	P	C	X	L	Q	U	B	B	D	A	D	R	U	X	E
Q	K	B	O	I	E	O	G	V	D	C	J	F	E	R	S	R	H	D	L
O	R	H	P	I	X	N	Y	G	R	C	O	Q	U	S	Y	N	B	I	Y
G	E	E	R	K	P	J	V	S	J	O	N	C	J	O	T	K	N	H	H
R	N	G	L	Z	E	G	F	S	C	A	U	S	A	L	I	T	Y	S	V
A	N	E	V	A	C	P	A	I	D	X	J	X	B	J	P	T	Z	U	X
H	B	Z	V	S	T	Q	M	G	C	R	Z	A	M	C	X	V	I	R	Z
R	M	V	K	X	E	E	R	V	O	V	W	G	U	Z	U	Z	C	U	G
D	M	B	F	N	D	K	D	F	G	H	N	Z	X	O	J	M	A	S	H

23. Pharmacovigilance (ii)

A	X	P	A	R	G	I	Z	J	S	E	P	G	P	D	P	L	A	L	O
R	P	X	M	B	P	J	E	C	W	L	W	O	L	N	X	T	D	Y	H
D	O	D	E	U	V	N	K	M	E	E	U	I	S	J	S	N	S	P	U
F	A	O	L	M	C	I	O	M	S	T	M	L	N	S	Y	Z	U	N	G
Z	J	L	W	S	G	B	W	S	I	B	G	R	Y	L	I	C	W	N	M
K	M	Q	S	E	K	I	X	Y	B	K	U	X	E	D	Q	B	N	N	B
N	Z	V	P	V	B	P	U	M	K	Z	D	T	I	O	U	L	L	B	J
E	F	A	F	E	K	C	J	G	S	G	I	O	Y	J	O	R	V	Y	P
R	K	D	T	R	F	G	H	J	D	N	E	I	L	O	Y	Y	K	R	F
C	Z	Z	U	E	J	R	X	M	I	H	G	B	D	K	L	V	P	O	X
N	G	P	N	X	F	U	C	F	O	F	M	Q	V	B	J	K	J	S	R
S	X	Y	R	Y	V	L	E	M	N	F	J	E	A	Y	W	C	E	A	R
F	D	L	E	K	C	D	Y	W	G	G	E	B	D	D	E	Y	H	L	E
Y	S	Y	L	K	L	P	U	W	Y	F	O	F	W	W	C	E	K	D	R
R	T	S	A	T	A	U	O	O	X	R	G	D	C	D	A	Q	E	Y	A
I	T	V	T	U	D	W	Q	L	P	E	R	V	U	C	D	T	R	T	V
F	U	G	E	S	Y	D	U	Q	D	R	X	A	V	T	F	K	C	A	U
H	A	V	D	P	E	F	E	A	Q	P	L	F	W	H	S	O	X	H	N
I	X	K	T	L	V	M	O	D	E	R	A	T	E	S	P	S	U	R	V
K	J	Z	L	T	Z	S	Y	J	V	W	H	B	N	E	G	K	J	Q	G

24. Clinical Trial Documents

T	W	I	E	H	M	E	L	D	V	M	V	L	H	N	D	G	N	G	V
I	P	N	R	M	O	Y	C	Q	J	N	P	F	H	O	F	R	F	T	R
I	R	D	C	E	K	H	J	A	K	R	K	C	T	A	Z	F	I	L	L
Z	V	E	Q	E	Y	P	J	S	V	Y	T	N	X	G	R	Y	A	L	T
P	P	M	P	R	X	O	A	U	U	G	X	I	W	F	I	V	G	F	I
K	G	N	Q	U	J	E	I	T	S	R	X	M	K	W	O	I	P	U	U
Z	X	I	D	C	X	C	I	S	I	U	Z	B	E	R	D	B	R	K	A
P	R	F	K	O	W	C	O	R	L	E	F	Q	P	L	D	N	E	J	K
U	I	I	V	R	M	G	R	S	B	E	N	P	C	F	F	U	F	A	O
C	B	C	H	G	K	T	S	F	Z	A	A	T	M	S	L	S	A	B	I
Y	O	A	W	U	E	V	Z	L	A	Y	P	X	D	O	P	A	I	O	J
F	V	T	F	Y	F	L	W	F	R	B	J	P	C	I	A	R	X	M	N
I	S	I	A	U	T	X	E	O	H	R	P	O	R	N	A	C	N	Q	P
R	P	O	N	W	V	H	T	N	L	B	T	T	T	O	A	R	G	W	Y
I	V	N	G	U	T	A	F	X	S	O	V	W	O	Z	V	X	I	J	N
E	C	A	W	Q	L	V	G	F	R	Y	L	D	E	N	K	A	F	E	F
U	N	D	O	U	G	O	M	P	X	R	S	C	H	M	C	O	L	Z	S
U	X	V	G	Z	V	T	C	I	N	S	U	R	A	N	C	E	K	Z	E
H	E	E	Y	B	H	H	O	O	D	N	D	R	D	V	T	F	P	Y	B
C	R	Y	I	D	M	I	O	Z	Q	D	L	S	G	E	H	S	Q	A	N

25. Source Documents

R	N	U	M	I	C	R	O	F	I	C	H	E	S	F	B	S	K	E	L
E	C	G	F	Y	D	G	Z	Y	E	P	D	K	Y	U	D	D	Z	L	N
C	W	D	Y	Y	W	A	J	C	S	X	P	F	X	R	V	K	M	G	G
L	A	I	B	U	G	E	U	H	O	R	R	G	O	W	E	U	I	G	Z
I	U	P	A	P	O	V	D	U	H	O	W	C	Z	X	R	R	C	G	Z
N	M	E	H	R	T	Y	M	H	P	U	E	T	S	S	T	S	R	M	X
I	F	W	U	Z	X	H	Z	W	F	R	Z	W	L	F	E	B	O	Z	R
C	R	W	U	S	C	O	A	H	Y	Q	R	W	X	I	L	V	F	E	A
A	P	J	I	X	J	O	I	C	V	Q	J	U	R	V	A	O	I	L	Y
L	O	L	T	J	Q	P	A	N	I	Q	J	A	O	R	B	S	L	Y	S
C	O	R	Q	P	L	M	Z	W	W	L	I	D	C	Y	R	V	M	B	G
H	T	M	A	K	R	C	J	M	R	D	B	R	S	R	E	F	S	K	V
A	S	U	V	A	R	C	W	C	T	A	W	N	N	X	P	I	C	O	Y
R	F	U	H	Z	G	E	D	C	R	Q	A	S	K	A	O	B	E	D	M
T	B	P	G	K	N	Y	E	Y	B	C	E	B	J	U	R	U	N	T	O
S	D	G	C	K	M	J	U	J	S	T	U	A	F	G	T	U	K	O	V
M	H	R	U	X	B	K	M	T	D	F	M	C	H	H	S	O	T	Z	L
Q	F	R	Q	U	R	C	C	B	H	D	Z	V	J	Y	K	N	V	Q	E
Y	M	X	S	P	H	O	S	P	I	T	A	L	R	E	C	O	R	D	S
T	O	T	I	K	T	R	R	X	M	G	J	U	O	F	U	A	S	C	N

26. Vulnerable Population

O J M X X O F G S A F B U W T N N C D X
D I P I N U R S I N G S T U D E N T S P
U A Z X P V G A W P I M T G W S V S A Q
K W W L A G A M P I N G U Q T M N M R T
W E M M G V X V G S D A H N K O R I M X
A B X E G W G Y D A F E E H S J E N E L
U U Y R D U G A O Z I D Z R R V U O D U
Z Z M C E I M R L T U N E R Z F W R F J
A M P B D O C J O T D P D L Z D Z I O Y
X K A N N Y K A S W D F Y X D S F T R Q
V R L A H E S Y L E I E F K X D F Y C K
U J C E B E C X Y S Y M Y W Y K E G E Q
G P V S E A H O D S T R O E V S X R M I
V Z W O M Y L J H Z S U E Q G W R O E Q
H U U R W P B F M L V Y D F H Y W U M R
X G A Y M S L I I U N F V E U Y K P B H
I H C E Z G H P N M A C O V N G V S E C
P M N D L L E W O R F X P Y Q T E U R T
X U H J N C I B R D P W N Q B X S E S K
N J Z P B K R P S P R I S O N E R S S Z

27. Investigator Site Evaluation/Qualification

Y	X	X	C	P	A	T	H	U	B	M	B	E	D	D	A	J	K	R	N
Q	S	D	V	N	A	Z	S	X	K	N	H	S	O	D	Y	S	F	O	J
C	C	O	Y	W	I	T	S	M	J	E	S	Y	H	K	C	U	I	J	R
S	S	S	U	C	R	J	I	K	F	E	L	G	O	O	M	T	K	X	E
V	Y	T	O	R	B	F	S	E	I	H	Y	K	Z	A	A	T	J	W	E
K	I	D	U	L	C	Z	V	R	N	B	Y	X	I	C	X	C	G	U	X
G	O	Q	S	D	P	E	O	B	R	T	H	Z	I	M	Y	N	H	D	F
X	T	H	T	B	Y	T	D	O	D	Y	P	F	F	V	A	C	T	P	C
J	R	W	Q	W	A	T	L	O	H	C	I	O	N	X	I	Y	B	H	C
Q	G	Y	F	R	T	V	E	M	C	L	B	B	O	W	Y	I	E	X	E
Z	D	A	O	H	E	W	G	A	A	U	S	B	I	L	R	C	S	A	P
S	K	B	N	Z	W	D	E	U	M	U	M	S	S	Y	O	T	S	G	N
K	A	M	O	B	J	X	Q	K	V	P	X	E	N	D	N	A	U	Y	Z
L	G	S	X	J	J	I	U	H	T	H	H	Z	N	F	E	H	E	S	G
S	F	G	Q	C	P	O	R	H	K	L	K	A	H	T	N	U	S	T	Y
W	O	U	I	R	M	Z	E	H	I	F	Q	X	R	C	S	Q	J	O	T
A	K	E	D	C	T	U	K	H	Q	W	W	M	Z	M	I	Z	V	R	Q
I	N	F	R	A	S	T	R	U	C	T	U	R	E	Q	A	B	X	A	T
P	G	J	Q	Y	O	T	S	D	X	K	S	Y	D	I	O	C	D	G	Q
P	F	A	C	I	L	I	T	Y	V	I	S	I	T	C	E	S	Y	E	E

28. Essential Trial Documents (Before the Clinical Phase of the Trial Commences)

L	I	N	S	U	R	A	N	C	E	S	T	A	T	E	M	E	N	T	G
S	A	W	L	M	Y	G	O	Y	E	A	P	V	L	A	J	L	X	T	S
I	D	V	S	U	S	A	K	H	C	I	N	K	M	G	E	I	L	E	Q
G	V	Q	H	O	S	I	U	D	P	U	F	G	K	W	C	A	G	K	I
N	E	I	I	K	E	M	G	V	W	Q	R	S	N	O	V	N	T	X	R
E	R	I	R	C	P	U	Y	N	A	T	U	M	K	O	A	F	M	M	B
D	T	G	B	B	E	V	K	L	E	I	J	J	R	R	Z	F	F	Q	C
A	I	T	A	K	J	B	N	E	K	D	I	P	E	P	T	B	H	M	O
G	S	S	P	Y	Y	Y	S	X	H	U	P	C	X	N	O	Y	O	A	M
R	E	T	P	D	H	H	G	N	I	A	N	R	J	G	J	T	S	Q	P
E	M	D	R	W	V	G	P	Q	Y	E	O	W	O	X	G	W	Q	Q	O
E	E	V	O	Y	B	F	N	R	R	I	Z	T	Y	T	Y	N	E	B	S
M	N	S	V	M	C	F	O	E	P	B	B	X	F	L	O	L	Z	B	I
E	T	B	A	I	K	T	F	U	J	G	F	I	H	R	U	C	L	R	T
N	E	O	L	M	A	E	X	I	I	N	I	Z	F	K	G	W	O	Q	I
T	O	F	B	L	R	M	U	G	Q	E	S	G	M	T	S	Z	A	L	O
S	F	J	U	B	T	H	B	D	R	X	N	X	Q	C	Y	U	N	T	N
Q	W	G	A	O	A	D	R	I	N	A	W	S	D	F	S	Y	B	G	M
V	E	L	Q	F	T	G	U	N	R	B	P	C	E	E	A	E	N	Q	Q
R	Q	W	O	D	P	I	X	U	J	F	I	N	J	L	B	R	K	Q	V

29. Essential Trial Documents (During the Clinical Conduct of the Trial)

P	A	C	I	C	O	M	P	L	E	T	E	D	C	R	F	F	V	K	H
R	L	O	P	G	A	B	Z	A	X	X	Q	A	H	U	T	A	R	V	V
O	U	L	A	J	S	J	F	B	C	G	L	O	G	X	W	W	S	X	S
T	V	K	C	D	I	V	P	X	Q	B	H	R	F	T	D	G	O	E	K
O	M	N	C	Q	G	C	M	M	X	C	Q	V	U	K	O	P	U	U	P
C	C	X	O	S	N	M	D	S	X	B	L	X	G	L	K	F	R	E	C
O	M	B	U	P	E	A	Q	A	V	Z	Z	P	T	Z	V	X	C	T	R
L	D	M	N	U	D	W	R	H	M	A	G	N	E	B	Y	K	E	V	Z
A	C	J	T	S	I	V	R	H	I	E	E	X	I	R	F	R	D	C	C
M	I	P	A	E	C	R	I	J	U	M	N	Q	R	S	O	K	O	N	A
E	G	H	B	T	D	N	Y	B	L	W	T	D	F	N	S	V	C	S	E
N	Q	R	I	Z	M	E	N	O	U	U	I	B	M	E	F	U	U	C	R
D	E	W	L	W	H	U	R	F	B	P	N	K	S	E	C	E	M	H	U
M	W	Z	I	Z	K	N	M	K	X	E	D	J	G	Z	N	W	E	O	P
E	F	T	T	Z	E	N	M	U	D	Q	K	A	G	W	Z	T	N	R	N
N	L	E	Y	Y	G	H	E	T	X	K	Q	T	T	Q	J	F	T	G	W
T	X	S	L	X	K	U	G	P	Y	H	B	T	O	E	W	W	S	X	K
D	T	M	O	N	I	T	O	R	I	N	G	R	E	P	O	R	T	S	A
U	F	X	G	P	N	E	H	E	U	J	U	E	B	L	U	Q	F	S	Q
Q	J	W	S	A	S	C	R	E	E	N	I	N	G	L	O	G	O	Q	Z

30. Essential Trial Documents (After Completion or Termination of the Trial)

S	U	B	J	E	C	T	I	D	C	O	D	E	L	I	S	T	E	Z	E
F	I	N	A	L	P	A	Y	M	E	N	T	R	E	C	O	R	D	G	I
V	I	P	A	C	C	O	U	N	T	A	B	I	L	I	T	Y	N	S	A
Y	N	M	I	A	R	C	H	I	V	E	L	O	C	A	T	I	O	N	U
V	D	P	J	P	J	T	H	X	H	G	D	B	B	S	T	M	X	W	D
F	P	Z	Z	A	D	Y	X	A	X	A	D	K	S	R	A	B	D	F	I
N	Y	G	S	G	Y	E	Q	B	W	D	T	V	O	C	S	S	P	I	T
W	I	M	N	J	U	V	S	H	I	B	D	P	N	Y	Z	D	B	T	C
W	C	C	R	J	G	U	U	T	D	L	E	C	P	W	F	S	V	S	E
I	N	E	F	L	N	E	T	F	R	R	N	I	S	H	Z	R	U	F	R
X	X	U	O	I	J	K	C	N	Y	U	V	J	P	F	Y	E	M	A	T
W	A	Q	R	Q	C	T	H	R	M	C	C	S	S	L	D	V	Y	S	I
V	S	I	T	E	C	L	O	S	E	O	U	T	R	E	P	O	R	T	F
P	X	B	C	W	A	T	U	R	U	S	R	Y	I	F	L	V	I	Q	I
V	J	N	S	F	A	C	Z	C	W	M	Z	I	R	O	S	R	Y	I	C
T	L	C	Y	L	J	H	B	F	V	M	U	H	F	W	N	H	Q	P	A
U	M	W	U	B	O	S	I	G	N	E	D	C	S	R	Z	L	W	E	T
G	Z	G	W	A	U	K	E	R	I	P	M	U	G	K	K	U	O	I	E
G	E	R	F	Q	B	G	U	T	R	I	B	J	L	U	B	C	J	G	T
R	D	R	M	G	B	Z	I	R	B	R	E	P	O	R	T	I	N	G	S

31. Clinical Trial Terminologies

B	C	C	B	Y	J	A	E	U	I	K	H	S	O	Y	P	Y	I	C	N
O	L	Y	Y	K	W	S	D	V	W	R	D	V	A	O	I	F	N	A	P
K	I	I	Y	P	M	L	T	R	C	A	N	W	Q	G	V	O	S	X	D
U	S	T	N	Q	X	Z	H	P	A	N	O	N	Y	Y	G	X	P	F	F
R	I	R	N	D	Z	A	Z	D	R	D	V	V	N	Z	Y	K	E	N	G
T	K	R	P	U	I	H	H	D	E	O	J	X	R	B	T	G	C	S	E
R	R	O	R	O	C	N	B	E	P	M	R	J	Z	V	W	C	T	X	R
I	S	C	Y	X	W	H	G	F	O	I	R	D	I	T	Z	C	I	Y	I
A	P	J	B	K	K	B	Q	J	E	Z	U	V	W	S	R	G	O	L	X
L	C	S	S	R	K	M	S	Z	Z	A	U	C	H	Y	H	U	N	D	C
S	B	N	C	H	Y	P	Z	N	N	T	H	O	Z	A	J	F	V	J	X
I	O	U	Y	F	K	R	T	N	O	I	J	M	J	T	U	J	P	K	C
T	U	S	H	Y	O	O	E	X	K	O	N	P	K	V	V	Z	J	N	K
E	W	I	B	L	O	K	A	G	A	N	A	L	P	P	C	S	L	G	T
G	D	S	N	S	J	P	C	W	F	L	Z	I	Z	T	R	U	A	C	L
G	S	O	U	R	C	E	D	A	T	A	X	A	N	T	O	R	Y	E	N
R	G	H	G	O	Z	F	C	I	J	U	E	N	K	P	Y	S	S	I	T
O	A	O	V	W	O	X	V	M	M	R	O	C	Y	O	N	F	G	J	L
H	Q	G	E	C	X	C	Y	X	S	R	X	E	K	Y	L	J	W	X	V
L	Z	Q	W	A	U	D	I	T	T	R	A	I	L	B	G	E	E	X	M

4

Odd-One-Out

In this section you will find items pertaining to **15** clinical trial elements/activities/processes. You have to identify the Odd-One-Out for each element/activity/process and mention it in the empty box provided at the bottom of each exercise.

Scoring: Excellent (able to solve ≥13 exercises); Very Good (≥12 to <13 exercises); Good (≥10 to <12 exercises); Satisfactory (≥7 to <10 exercises); Unsatisfactory (<7 exercises).

1. Essential Clinical Trial Documents

- Protocol
- Investigator's Brochure
- Case Report Form
- Clinical Study Report
- Informed Consent Document
- Informed Consent Document Translations
- Import License
- CV of Investigator
- Insurance
- Marketing Authorization
- Certificate of Analysis
- Contract/Agreements
- Export License
- Source Documents
- Regulatory Approval
- IRB/IEC/EC Approval
- Advertisement
- Investigational Product Accountability Log

Marketing Authorization

2. Drug Development Process

- Phase 0
- Phase I
- Phase II
- Phase III
- Phase IV
- Drug Launch

3. Clinical Trial Documents Required for Regulatory Approval

- Protocol
- Informed Consent Document
- Translations of Informed Consent Document
- Investigator's Brochure
- Case Report Form
- Investigator Undertaking
- CV of Investigator
- Data Management Plan
- Financial Agreement

4. Clinical Trial Stakeholders

- Sponsor
- Investigator
- Sub Investigator
- Clinical Research Coordinator
- Nurse
- Regulatory Agencies
- Contract Research Organization
- Site Management Organization

5. Responsibilities of Investigator

- Patient Care
- Patient Counseling
- GCP Compliance
- Safety Reporting to Regulatory Authorities
- Protocol Compliance
- Randomization
- Safety Reporting to Ethics Committee
- Case Report Form Completion
- Investigational Product Accountability
- Documentation of Violations/Deviations
- Site Close out

6. Responsibilities of Sponsor

- Development of Protocol
- Safety Reporting to Ethics Committee
- Safety Reporting to Regulatory Authorities
- Investigational Product Accountability
- Procurement of Import License
- Procurement of Export License
- Contracts/Agreements
- Clinical Trial Supplies Management
- Auditing
- Clinical Trial Monitoring
- Site Close out

7. Responsibilities of Regulatory Agencies

- Approval of Essential Clinical Trial Documents
- Inspection of Investigator Site, Sponsor, Ethics Committee
- Ensuring Compliance to GCP and Applicable Regulatory Guidelines
- Procurement of Import / Export License
- Review and Approval of Amendments
- Review of Progress of the Clinical Trial
- Protection of the Rights and Safety of Research Subjects

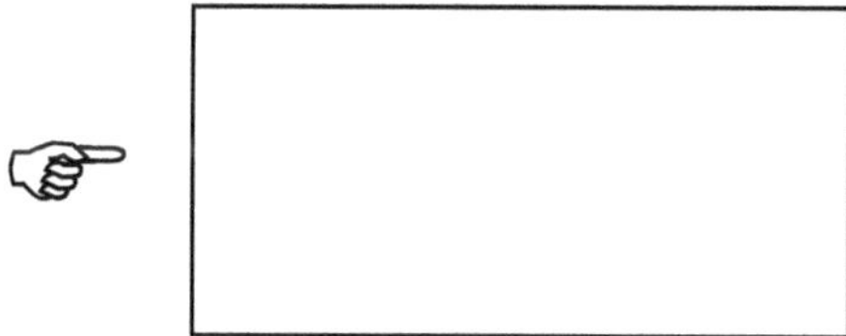

8. Activities Performed by Monitor during a Clinical Trial Monitoring Visit

- Check for Protocol Compliance
- Informed Consent Document Review
- Serious Adverse Event Review/Reporting
- Investigational Product Accountability
- Case Report Form Completion
- Case Report Forms Retrieval
- Meeting with Investigator and Study Team
- Check for GCP Compliance
- Source Data Verification
- Documentation of Deviation and Actionables
- Check for Regulatory Compliance

9. ICH-GCP Required Elements for Informed Consent Document

- Research Study
- Voluntary Participation
- Treatment Procedure
- Duration
- Alternative Therapy
- Risk and Benefit
- Compensation
- Anticipated Payments
- Non Confidentiality
- Sponsor Details
- Regulatory Details

10. Criterias for a Serious Adverse Event

- Death
- Life Threatening
- Permanent Disability
- Congenital Anomaly
- Accident leading to Hospitalization
- Adverse Event of Severe Nature
- Prolonged Hospitalization

11. Agenda Topics for Investigator's Training Meeting

- Study Protocol
- Informed Consent Document Administration Process
- GCP Guidelines
- Role of Monitor
- Case Report Form Completion
- Publication Policy
- Data Validation Plan
- Investigational Product Administration
- Safety Reporting
- Study Timelines

12. Essential Elements of Site Feasibility Assessment

- Investigator Qualification
- Recruitment Potential of the Investigator
- Availability of Study Staff
- Review of Signed ICF
- Laboratory Facilities
- Storage and Archival Facility
- Diagnostic Services

13. Project Milestones Planning

- Development of Essential Trial Documents
- Regulatory Approval Date
- Ethics Approval Date
- Investigator Training Meeting
- First Patient Visit
- Last Patient Enter Treatment
- Last Patient Visit
- Data Lock
- Site Closure
- Clinical Study Report (CSR) Preparation
- Trial Close-out
- Archival
- Drug Launch

14. Drug Regulatory Agencies

- FDA
- EMEA
- DCGI
- TGA
- MHRA
- MEDWATCH
- CDSCO
- ANVISA

15. Responsibilities of Ethics Committee (EC)

- Protection of Rights, Safety and Well Being of Trial Subjects
- Review of Essential Trial Documents for Granting Approvals
- Continuing Review of Ongoing Trials at least once per Year
- Review of Interim Analysis Data to Advise the Study Sponsors whether to Continue or Terminate the Trial
- Meeting the Quorum Requirements
- Composition, Function and Operations as per the Applicable Regulatory Requirements
- Maintaining the Minutes of the EC Meetings
- Retention of All Relevant Records for the Specified Period of Time

☞

5

Process Flows

In this section you will find **20** Process Flows based on clinical research topics. You have to identify the missing step(s)/element(s) and mention it at the relevant place(s).

Scoring: Excellent (able to solve ≥18 exercises); Very Good (≥16 to <18 exercises); Good (≥14 to <16 exercises); Satisfactory (≥10 to <14 exercises); Unsatisfactory (<10 exercises).

1. Drug Discovery Process

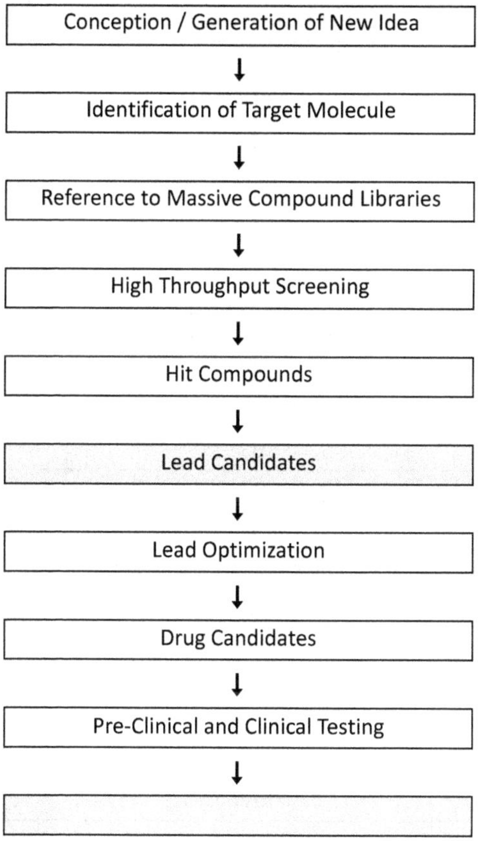

Conception / Generation of New Idea

↓

Identification of Target Molecule

↓

Reference to Massive Compound Libraries

↓

High Throughput Screening

↓

Hit Compounds

↓

Lead Candidates

↓

Lead Optimization

↓

Drug Candidates

↓

Pre-Clinical and Clinical Testing

↓

2. Drug Development Process

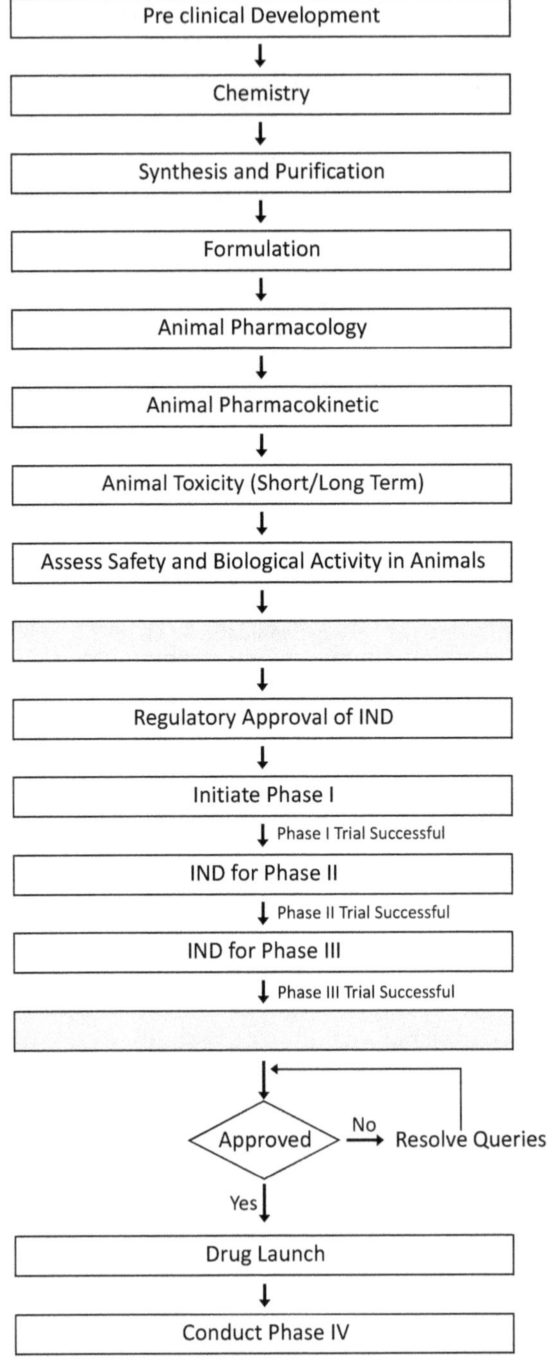

3. Trial Initiation

Project Feasibility Assessment and Planning of Milestones Dates (Sponsor)

↓

Constitution of Core Study Team (Sponsor)

↓

Development of Essential Trial Documents (Sponsor):

-
-
-
- Case Report Form
- Data Management Guidelines / Systems

↓

Financial Planning and Grants Allocation (Sponsor)

↓

Selection of CROs/Central Lab/ Data Management Center (Sponsor)

↓

Investigational Product Management:

- Inventory Planning (Investigational Agent / Comparator)
- Preparation and Manufacturing
-
-

↓

Site Selection (Sponsor/CRO) :

- Evaluation / Selection of Investigator Site(s)
- Appointment of Clinical Study Co-ordinator
- Resource Planning

↓

Preparation of Trial Binders (Sponsor/CRO):

- Project File
- Investigator File
- Training Binder
- Laboratory Manuals
- Translation of ICD and Relevant Documents in Vernacular Languages

↓

Contracts and Agreements (Sponsor / Investigator):

- Confidentiality Agreement
- Clinical Trial Agreement
- Protocol Acceptance and Investigator Undertaking
- Collection of CVs of Investigator Team, etc.

↓

↓

IRB/IEC/EC Approvals (Investigator)

↓

Regulatory Approvals (Sponsor/CRO)

↓

Investigator Site Training (Sponsor/CRO)

↓

Site Initiation (Sponsor/CRO)

4. Clinical Trial Project Management

Project Assignment

↓

Project Milestones Planning

↓

Development of Essential Documents (Protocol, IB, ICD, CRF)

↓

Investigator Site Selection, Contracts and Agreements

↓

IRB / EC / IEC Submission and Follow-up on Queries

↓

IRB / EC / IEC Approval

↓

Regulatory Submission and Follow-up on Queries

↓

Regulatory Approval

↓

Investigational Product Import / Procurement

↓

↓

First Patient Visit

↓

First Data to Database

↓

Last Patient Enter Treatment

↓

↓

Interim Data Lock (If applicable)

↓

Final Data Lock

↓

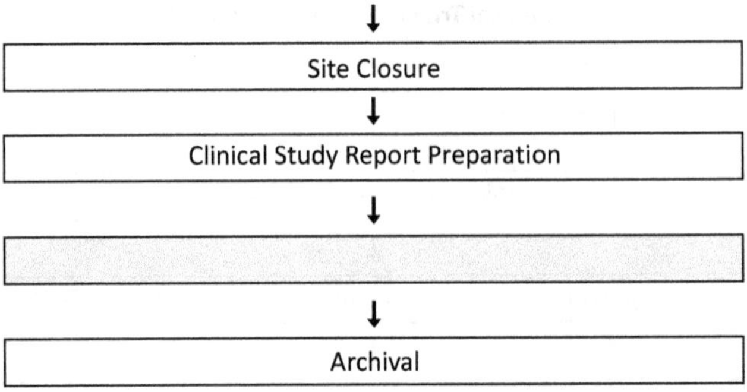

↓

Site Closure

↓

Clinical Study Report Preparation

↓

↓

Archival

5. Investigator Site Selection

Identification of Potential Investigational Site based on :

- Recruitment potential
- Investigator's Qualification and Past Clinical Trial Experience

Investigator Site Visit to :

- Discuss Study Design, Inclusion / Exclusion Criteria
- Assess Investigator Team, Team Qualification, Clinical Trial Exposure and Willingness
- Check Enrollment Status
-
- Check Source Data Documentation Practices
-
- Check Data Archival, Medical Record Retention at Site

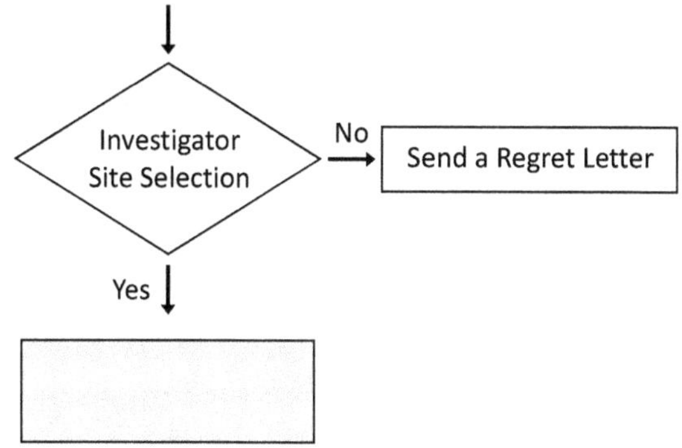

6. Organization Of Investigator's Training Meeting

Confirmation of Meeting Date / Time / Venue

↓

Logistics Management :
- Co-ordination with the Participating Investigators/Sites
- Necessary Travel Arrangements
- Preparation of Agenda and List of Participants
- Preparation of Training Binders/Presentations
- Audio Visual Equipments

↓

Conduct of Investigator's Training Meeting Covering Following Topics :
- Good Clinical Practices (GCP)
- Roles and Responsibilities
- Protocol
- Informed Consent Document (ICD) Process
- Serious Adverse Event (SAE) Process
- Source Documentation Practices
- Investigational Product (IP) Accountability
- Investigator Site File (ISF)
- CRF Completion and Data Management
- Study Timelines and Matrices

Obtaining Signature of all the Participants on the Sign-in Sheet/Log

↓

↓

7. Site Initiation

Pre Visit Activities:
- Planning of Site Initiation Visit
- Confirmation of Date and Time from the Site
- Necessary Travel Arrangements

On Site Activities:
- Meeting with Investigator / Staff to discuss:
    - Investigator / Staff Roles and Responsibilities
    - Facilities
    - Essential Trial Documents
    - Protocol, ICF Process, Randomization Procedures
    - SAE Process and Reporting Timelines
    - IP Storage and Accountability
    - Source Documentation
    - Study Timelines and Data Management
    - Audit/Inspection and Archival

Post Visit Activities:
-
-

8. Trial Conduct At Site

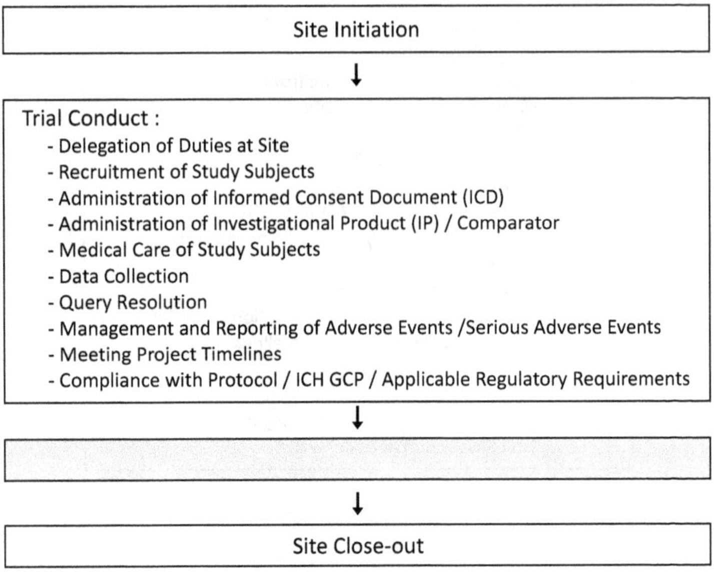

Site Initiation

↓

Trial Conduct :

- Delegation of Duties at Site
- Recruitment of Study Subjects
- Administration of Informed Consent Document (ICD)
- Administration of Investigational Product (IP) / Comparator
- Medical Care of Study Subjects
- Data Collection
- Query Resolution
- Management and Reporting of Adverse Events /Serious Adverse Events
- Meeting Project Timelines
- Compliance with Protocol / ICH GCP / Applicable Regulatory Requirements

↓

↓

Site Close-out

9. Process Flow For Obtaining Informed Consent Document (ICD) From Literates

Investigator or Designee Explains the Document to the Subject
↓
↓
Subject Asks the Queries (if any) to the Investigator or the Designee
↓
Subject Personally Signs and Dates the ICD in the Presence of Investigator or Designee (2 copies)
↓
↓
Subject Receives a Copy of the Signed ICD
↓
The Other Copy is Filed with the Study Documents at Site

10. Process Flow For Obtaining Informed Consent Document (ICD) From Illiterates

Investigator or Designee Explains the Document to the Subject in Presence of Subject's Legally Acceptable Representative

↓

Subject's Legally Acceptable Representative Personally Reads the ICD in Vernacular Language

↓

Subject's Legally Acceptable Representative Asks the Queries (if any) to the Investigator or the Designee

↓

↓

Subject Provides the Thumb Impression on Two Copies

↓

↓

Investigator or Designee Also Signs and Dates the ICD in the Presence of Subject and Subject's Legally Acceptable Representative

↓

Subject Receives a Copy of the Signed ICD

↓

The Other Copy is Filed with the Study Documents at Site

11. Process Flow For Obtaining Informed Consent Document (ICD) When Both Subject And Subject's Legally Acceptable Representative Are Illiterates

Investigator or Designee Explains the Document to the Subject (or Subject's Legally Acceptable Representative) in Presence of an Impartial Witness

↓

↓

Verbal Consent is Obtained from the Subject or Subject's Legally Acceptable Representative

↓

Subject or Subject's Legally Acceptable Representative Provides the Thumb Impression on Two Copies

↓

Impartial Witness Personally Signs and Dates the ICD in the Presence of Subject (or Subject's Legally Acceptable Representative) and the Investigator or Designee (2 Copies)

↓

Investigator or Designee also Signs and Dates the ICD in the Presence of Subject (or Subject's Legally Acceptable Representative) and Impartial Witness

↓

↓

The Other Copy is Filed with the Study Documents at Site

12. Translation Of Informed Consent Document (ICD) In Vernacular Language

Identification of Vernacular Language Requirements based on the Geographical Location of the Site

↓

Identification of a Translation Agency and Execution of Non Disclosure Agreement /Professional Service Agreement

↓

Forward the English ICD to the Translator

↓

↓

Forward the Vernacular Language ICD for Back Translation in English

↓

Back Translation of Vernacular Language ICD into English

↓

Validation of Back Translated ICD with the Original English ICD

↓

↓

Obtain Certificate of Translation

13. Serious Adverse Event (SAE) Reporting - Investigator's Responsibilities

SAE takes place at the Site

↓

Site Undertakes the Medical Management of the Event

↓

[illegible]

↓

Site Confirms the Receipt of SAE by the Sponsor

↓

Site Follow-up the Patient until the Event is Resolved

↓

Site Report Follow-up Information to the Sponsor within Stipulated Timeframe

↓

Site Resolves all the Queries Raised by the Sponsor's Pharmacovigilance Department

↓

[illegible]

↓

Site File all the Relevant Documents in the Respective Sections of the Site's Trial Binder/File

14. Serious Adverse Event (SAE) Reporting - Sponsor's Responsibilities

Sponsor's Designee Receives the SAE and Document the Date and Time of Receipt

↓

↓

Sponsor's Designee Discuss the Event with the Investigator and Assist in Ascertaining the Severity and Relatedness (if required)

↓

Sponsor's Designee Document all the Discussion/Clarification on SAE with the Site

↓

↓

Sponsor's Designee Share the Information with Other Trial Sites

↓

Sponsor's Designee Performs the Source Data Verification (SDV) of the SAE and all Discussion/Clarification During the Monitoring Visit

↓

Sponsor's Designee Performs the Review of IRB/IEC/EC Communications for Ensuring Compliance

↓

Sponsor's Designee Undertakes the Re-training of the Site on SAE Reporting (if required)

↓

Sponsor's Designee Files all the Relevant Documents in the Respective Section of the Trial Binder

15. Clinical Trial Monitoring

Pre Visit Activities:
- Planning of Monitoring Visit
- Confirmation of Date and Time of Visit
- Necessary Travel Arrangements

On Site Activities:
- Meeting with the Investigator/Research Team to Discuss the Progress of Trial
- Signature in Visitor's Log
- Review of :
    - Investigator Site File (ISF)
    - Source Document and Case Report Form (CRF)
    - •
    - Informed Consent Document (ICD)
    - Serious Adverse Events (SAEs)
    - •
    - Adequacy of facility and Study Team
- Collection of Case Report Form (CRF)
- -
- Closure Meeting with the Investigator/Team

Post Visit Activities:
- Preparation of Monitoring Visit Report
- Follow-up letter to the Site
- Resolution of Pending Issues (if any)

16. Management Of Protocol Deviation(s)/Violation(s)

Identification of Deviation/Violation

↓

Creation of Deviation File Note to Document :
- What Deviation has taken Place?
- Who is Responsible for the Deviation?
-
-

↓

Investigator's Signature on the Deviation File Note

↓

Signature of the Designated Personnel from the Sponsor on the Deviation File Note

↓

↓

Filing of Deviation/Violation in the Respective Section of Trial/Site Master File

17. Data Management Process (Paper CRF)

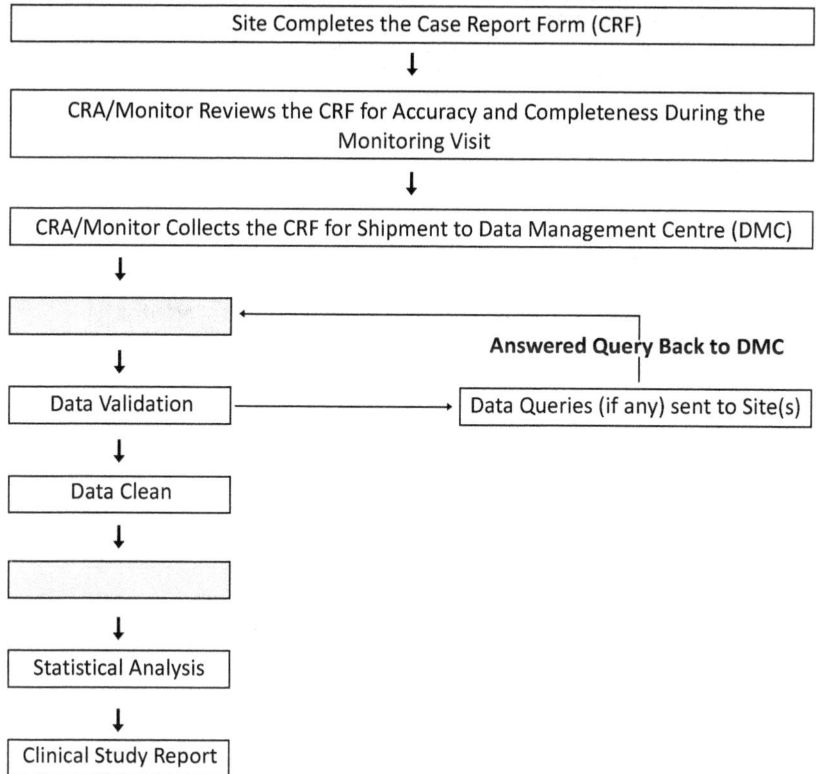

18. Site Close-Out

Pre Visit Activities:
- Notification to the Investigator for Site Close-out Visit
- Confirmation of Date and Time of Visit
- Necessary Travel Arrangements

On Site Activities:
- Review of Study Document and Finalization of all Pending Issues
-
- Return of Equipment/Study Supplies (if any)
-
- Discussion with Investigator about his/her Obligations of Archiving the Study Documents for the Specified Period of Time
-

Post Visit Activities:
- Preparation of Site Close-out Visit Report
- Resolution of Pending Issues (if any)

19. Trial Close-Out

Trial Completion/Termination/Suspension

↓

Site(s) Close-out

↓

↓

Review and Approval of Clinical Study Report from Participating Investigators

↓

Notification of Clinical Study Report to Regulatory Authorities

↓

↓

Archival

20. Regulatory Inspection Process (US-FDA)

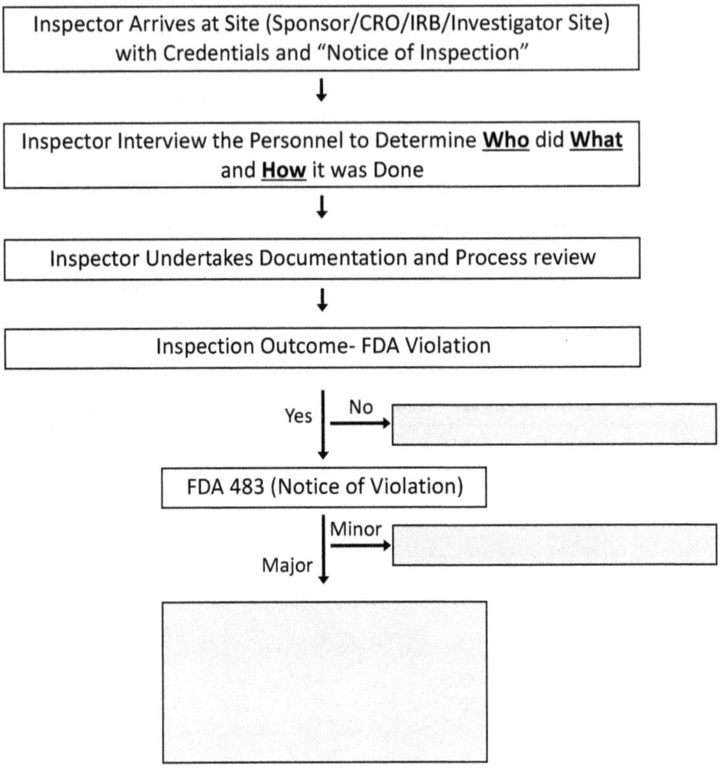

Inspector Arrives at Site (Sponsor/CRO/IRB/Investigator Site) with Credentials and "Notice of Inspection"

↓

Inspector Interview the Personnel to Determine **Who** did **What** and **How** it was Done

↓

Inspector Undertakes Documentation and Process review

↓

Inspection Outcome- FDA Violation

Yes ↓ | No →

FDA 483 (Notice of Violation)

Major ↓ | Minor →

www.ingramcontent.com/pod-product-compliance
Lightning Source LLC
Chambersburg PA
CBHW060405220326
41598CB00023B/3024

9788190827720